50 Cases in
Clinical Cardiology

50 Cases in Clinical Cardiology
A Problem Solving Approach

Atul Luthra MBBS MD DNB
Diplomate
National Board of Medicine
Physician and Cardiologist
New Delhi, India
www.atulluthra.in
atulluthra@sify.com

Foreword

JPS Sawhney

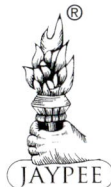

JAYPEE BROTHERS MEDICAL PUBLISHERS (P) LTD

New Delhi • London • Philadelphia • Panama

Jaypee Brothers Medical Publishers (P) Ltd.

Headquarters

Jaypee Brothers Medical Publishers (P) Ltd.
4838/24, Ansari Road, Daryaganj
New Delhi 110 002, India
Phone: +91-11-43574357
Fax: +91-11-43574314
Email: jaypee@jaypeebrothers.com

Overseas Offices

J.P. Medical Ltd.
83, Victoria Street, London
SW1H 0HW (UK)
Phone: +44-2031708910
Fax: +02-03-0086180
Email: info@jpmedpub.com

Jaypee-Highlights Medical
Publishers Inc.
City of Knowledge, Bld. 237, Clayton
Panama City, Panama
Phone: +1 507-301-0496
Fax: +1 507-301-0499
Email: cservice@jphmedical.com

Jaypee Medical Inc.
The Bourse
111, South Independence Mall East
Suite 835, Philadelphia
PA 19106, USA
Phone: + 1 267-519-9789
Email: joe.rusko@jaypeebrothers.com

Jaypee Brothers Medical
Publishers (P) Ltd.
17/1-B, Babar Road, Block-B
Shaymali, Mohammadpur
Dhaka-1207, Bangladesh
Mobile: +08801912003485
Email: jaypeedhaka@gmail.com

Jaypee Brothers Medical
Publishers (P) Ltd.
Bhotahity, Kathmandu, Nepal
Phone: +977-9741283608
Email: kathmandu@jaypeebrothers.com

Website: www.jaypeebrothers.com
Website: www.jaypeedigital.com

© 2014, Jaypee Brothers Medical Publishers

The views and opinions expressed in this book are solely those of the original contributor(s)/author(s) and do not necessarily represent those of editor(s) of the book.

All brand names and product names used in this book are trade names, service marks, trademarks or registered trademarks of their respective owners. The publisher is not associated with any product or vendor mentioned in this book.

Medical knowledge and practice change constantly. This book is designed to provide accurate, authoritative information about the subject matter in question. However, readers are advised to check the most current information available on procedures included and check information from the manufacturer of each product to be administered, to verify the recommended dose, formula, method and duration of administration, adverse effects and contraindications. It is the responsibility of the practitioner to take all appropriate safety precautions. Neither the publisher nor the author(s)/editor(s) assume any liability for any injury and/or damage to persons or property arising from or related to use of material in this book.

This book is sold on the understanding that the publisher is not engaged in providing professional medical services. If such advice or services are required, the services of a competent medical professional should be sought.

Every effort has been made where necessary to contact holders of copyright to obtain permission to reproduce copyright material. If any have been inadvertently overlooked, the publisher will be pleased to make the necessary arrangements at the first opportunity.

Inquiries for bulk sales may be solicited at: jaypee@jaypeebrothers.com

50 Cases in Clinical Cardiology: A Problem Solving Approach

First Edition: **2014**

ISBN 978-93-5152-110-5

Printed in India

Dedicated to
My Parents
Ms Prem Lata Luthra
and
Mr Prem Prakash Luthra
Who guide and bless me
from heaven

Foreword

With the widespread availability of sophisticated cutting-edge technology, the clinician's approach towards the diagnosis of heart disease has undergone a paradigm shift. These days, it is not uncommon for the patient to be wheeled into the ECHO-room or even the cath-lab, without anyone taking a medical history or even caring to place a stethoscope over the patient's precordium. This is not a good sign since history-taking along with clinical examination should continue to occupy their rightful place in the practice of bedside cardiology. Moreover, a wealth of information is available in simple diagnostic modalities such as the ECG and X-ray chest, which should be interpreted in the light of clinical data.

I must compliment Atul Luthra for this brilliant compilation of a wide variety of real-world clinical situations, encountered during the practice of cardiology. He has elegantly discussed each case and solved the clinical problem in a meticulous way. The section on discussion incorporates a bewildering array of high-quality ECG strips, X-ray films and ECHO images. Students preparing for their examinations, resident doctors working in cardiac units and clinicians involved in heart-care are bound to benefit from this book. I wish Atul and his excellent book, all the best.

JPS Sawhney
Chief of Clinical Cardiology
Chairman, Department of Cardiology
Sir Ganga Ram Hospital, New Delhi, India
www.preventivecardiology.in

Preface

Present-day cardiology is replete with a bewildering array of sophisticated investigative techniques, that have eclipsed the art of arriving at a diagnosis on the bedside of the patient. Yet, a relevant medical history and a meticulous physical examination are indispensable tools to mentally construct a plausible clinical diagnosis. Further, simple but informative investigations such as electrocardiography (ECG), chest radiography (X-ray) and echocardiography (ECHO), have withstood the test of time in clinical cardiology. Moreover, they are cost-effective in resource-sensitive settings and can be performed at the patient's bedside.

It gives me immense pleasure to proudly present *50 Cases in Clinical Cardiology: A Problem Solving Approach*, a compilation of real-world situations in clinical cardiology. Each case is introduced with a brief history and findings on physical examination. The clinical problem is then discussed analytically and ultimately solved with the aid of one or more simple bedside investigations. The case concludes with pertinent management issues along with some recent advances in diagnostics and therapeutics pertaining to that clinical entity. The text is suitably complemented by impressive illustrations of ECG strips, chest X-rays and ECHO images.

I have tried to incorporate most clinical situations encountered in heart clinics and cardiology ward-rounds, but there might be some omissions. Nevertheless, I sincerely hope that the wealth of clinical material on cardiac symptoms, physical signs and auscultatory findings, will rekindle the romance between the clinician and clinical cardiology. This book should be most useful for cardiology students preparing for examinations, resident doctors working in cardiac units as well as for physicians involved in the care of heart patients.

Atul Luthra

Acknowledgments

I am extremely grateful to:

- My teachers in school, who helped me to acquire good command over spoken and written English language.
- My lecturers and professors in medical college, who taught me the science and art of bedside cardiology.
- My heart patients, whose findings on clinical examination and results of investigations made me wiser.
- Learned authors of textbooks on clinical cardiology to which I referred liberally, while preparing the manuscript.
- My esteemed readers of earlier books, whose generous appreciation and constructive criticism keep me going.
- M/s Jaypee Brothers Medical Publishers (P) Ltd., New Delhi, India, who repose their unflinching faith in me and provide excellent editorial support.

Contents

Section 13: Cardiac Arrhythmias

Section 14: Coronary Artery Diseases

Congenital Heart Diseases

Ventricular
Septal Defect

Case Presentation

A 31-year old man was referred to the cardiologist by a general physician, for evaluation of a heart murmur. This young man had been denied a life insurance policy because the physician, empanelled by the insurance company, had incidentally noticed the murmur during medical examination. The man was normally very active and denied complaints of chest pain, breathlessness, palpitations or syncope. There was no history of cyanotic spells, joint pains or repeated chest infections during childhood and he regularly played cricket and football in school. However, the patient recollected that the doctor in the school medical room had noticed the murmur and made a note of it in his medical report.

On examination, the man was of average built and height and looked healthy. The pulse was 84 beats/min. and regular with no special character. The BP was 134/76 mm Hg in the right arm while sitting. There was no anemia, cyanosis or clinical sign of congestive heart failure. The apex beat was ill-sustained, heaving in nature and slightly displaced towards the axilla. There was a pansystolic murmur over the middle of the left sternal border with a S_3 sound in early diastole. The murmur did not radiate towards the axilla. There was no parasternal heave and the lower border of the liver was not palpable. The lung fields were clear.

CLINICAL DISCUSSION

From the history and physical examination, this asymptomatic young man had a parasternal pansystolic murmur. Typical causes of a pansystolic murmur are mitral regurgitation, ventricular septal defect and tricuspid regurgitation. Sometimes, tight coarctation of aorta or a patent ductus arteriosus with pulmonary hypertension can also produce a pansystolic murmur but these murmurs are usually located at the upper left sternal edge. The murmur of mitral regurgitation radiates towards the axilla while the murmur of tricuspid regurgitation is usually associated with engorged neck veins and an enlarged pulsatile liver.

ECG of the patient showed biphasic RS complexes in the mid-precordial leads. X-ray chest showed mild cardiomegaly with minimal signs of pulmonary congestion. On ECHO, the left ventricle was normal in size with normal ejection fraction. A signal drop-out was noticed in the mid-portion of the interventricular

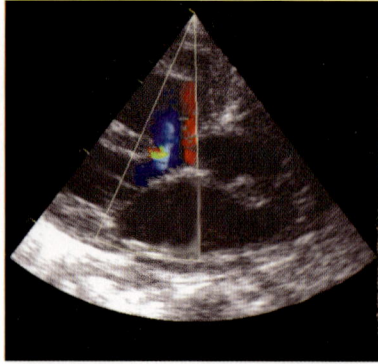

Figure 1.1: Color flow map extending from left ventricle to right ventricle

septum. There was no abnormality of the cardiac valves and the estimated pulmonary artery pressure was normal. On color Doppler, an abnormal flow map was observed extending from the left ventricle to the right ventricle (Fig. 1.1), with a high velocity jet on continuous wave Doppler. Therefore, the definite diagnosis in this case is ventricular septal defect (VSD).

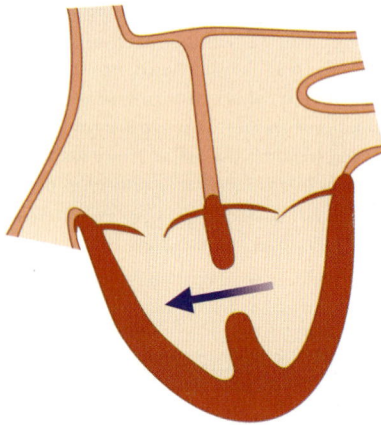

Figure 1.2: Ventricular septal defect

In VSD, a breach in the continuity of the interventricular septum creates a left-to-right shunt between the ventricles (Fig. 1.2). This congenital cardiac defect occurs due to complexity of embryological development of the septum, which has a membranous and a muscular portion. Most (80%) VSDs occur at the junction of these sections and are termed as perimembranous VSD (Fig. 1.3). Some VSDs occur in the muscular section (muscular VSD) and may be multiple (sieve-like). Rare varieties of VSD are endocardial cushion defects (supracristal VSD) and outlet septal defect (subpulmonic VSD) (Table 1.1).

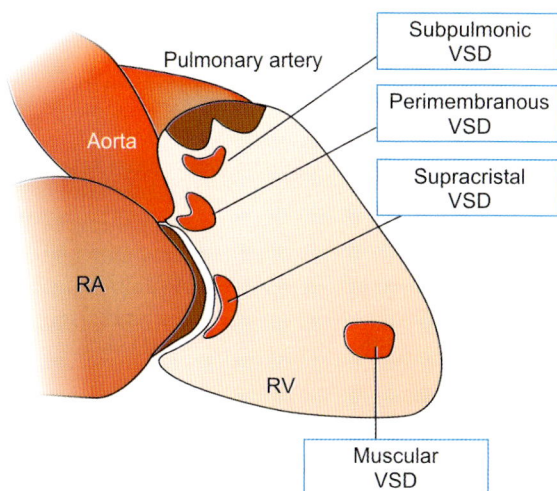

Figure 1.3: Various locations of ventricular septal defect (VSD)
RA: Right atrium; RV: Right ventricle

Table 1.1: Types of ventricular septal defect
• Perimembranous VSD
• Subpulmonic VSD
• Supracristal VSD
• Muscular VSD

A small VSD (Maladie de Roger) generates a loud pansystolic murmur in a localized area on the precordium. The murmur is located in the upper parasternal area in outlet VSD and in the mid-portion in perimembranous VSD. A muscular VSD produces a short systolic murmur since the defect shuts off during muscle contraction in later systole. This murmur is located over the lower parasternal area. A large VSD with elevated right ventricular pressure that equals left ventricular pressure (bidirectional shunt) is also associated with an early systolic murmur. Therefore, there is no correlation between the length or intensity of the murmur and the size of the VSD.

A large shunt may be accompanied by a diastolic flow murmur and a S_3 sound, due to torrential flow across the mitral valve. The S_2 is widely split due to early aortic valve closure. On ECHO, signal drop-out is not observed if the VSD is too small (<3 mm size) or muscular in location. The width of the colour flow map approximates the VSD size. On Doppler, high flow velocity indicates a small VSD. The flow velocity is low if the VSD is large and the shunt is bidirectional.

VSD is the commonest form of congenital acyanotic heart disease and accounts for 25% of all cardiac malformations. VSD may occur in isolation or as part of a complex constellation of congenital cardiac abnormalities. Aortic regurgitation may be associated due to lack of support to the aortic valve in perimembranous

VSD. Complications of VSD in childhood are growth retardation and repeated chest infections. Reversal of shunt can occur later in life when pulmonary pressure exceeds the systemic pressure. Endocarditis can follow any non-cardiac surgical procedure.

MANAGEMENT ISSUES

Large sized VSDs allow large volumes of left-to-right shunt and usually present in childhood with failure to thrive, breathlessness and recurrent respiratory infections. They can lead to pulmonary hypertension, right heart failure and ultimately reversal of shunt (right-to-left). This is designated as the Eisenmenger's syndrome. Such VSDs are usually closed in childhood to avoid complications and before the Eisenmenger's syndrome has developed.

Medium sized VSDs are associated with a moderate sized shunt. The shunt is large enough to cause breathlessness, but not enough to cause pulmonary hypertension and shunt reversal. Such patients do reasonably well during childhood, but may become progressively symptomatic as left ventricular compliance declines with age and pulmonary venous congestion develops. Such VSDs are usually closed in adulthood, to avoid the development of heart failure.

Small sized VSDs do not cause significant shunting and are often asymptomatic. Some of them may close as the child grows older. Those that do not close spontaneously are closed by intervention for reasons other than the shunt. These reasons are development of endocarditis or associated significant aortic regurgitation (Table 1.2).

Table 1.2: Indications for surgical closure of VSD
• Large-sized VSD with volume overload (pulmonary to systemic flow ratio >2:1)
• Medium-sized VSD with congestive symptoms without pulmonary hypertension
• Small-sized VSD without congestive symptoms with endocarditis or aortic regurgitation

RECENT ADVANCES

The last decade or two have witnessed remarkable progress in the percutaneous techniques for closure of ventricular septal defects, thus avoiding the risks associated with open heart surgery. Although transesophageal echocardiography (TEE) generally suffices to guide the deployment of the closure device, intracardiac ultrasound provides more accurate assessment. Sonography can provide vital information pertaining to the location and size of the defect and the rim around it, so as to facilitate proper device selection and placement.

Atrial Septal Defect

Case Presentation

A 36-year old woman was referred to a physician by a gynecologist, for preoperative assessment prior to elective hysterectomy. The patient had multiple uterine fibroids on ultrasonography and complained of excessive bleeding during menstruation. For the past 6 months, she had been complaining of exertional dyspnea and fatigue, which were attributed to anemia as a result of blood loss. She denied complaints of chest pain, palpitations or dizziness. There was no history of cyanotic spells, joint pains or recurrent respiratory infections during her childhood. The patient was married, had 2 sons aged 11 and 9 years and she had never been hospitalized for any major illness or surgical procedure.

On examination there was mild anemia but no cyanosis, icterus or sign of congestive heart failure. The pulse was 90 beats/min. regular, with a BP of 136/80 mm Hg in the right arm. The apex beat was normal in location with a sustained left parasternal heave on palpation. The S_1 was normal with a loud P_2; no S_3 or S_4 sound was heard. The S_2 components namely A_2 and P_2 were widely spaced and the time gap between them did not increase further during inspiration. A short systolic murmur was heard over the upper left sternal border. The murmur was not preceded by an ejection click or accompanied by a palpable thrill and did not radiate to the neck. The lung fields were clear on auscultation.

CLINICAL DISCUSSION

From the history and physical examination, this young woman had effort intolerance with an ejection murmur in the pulmonary area. Typical causes of such a murmur are innocent hemic murmur (Still's murmur), pulmonary valve stenosis, pulmonary hypertension and atrial septal defect. The murmur of pulmonary stenosis may be preceded by an ejection click and accompanied by a palpable thrill. The P_2 component of S_2 is muffled and the splitting between A_2 and P_2 is wide, but widens further during inspiration. An innocent hemic murmur is not associated with a loud P_2 or wide splitting of S_2. Pulmonary hypertension of any etiology can produce a systolic murmur with loud P_2 but wide fixed splitting of S_2 is only a feature of atrial septal defect.

ECG of the patient showed sinus rhythm with incomplete right bundle branch block and a rightward QRS axis. X-ray chest showed enlarged right-sided

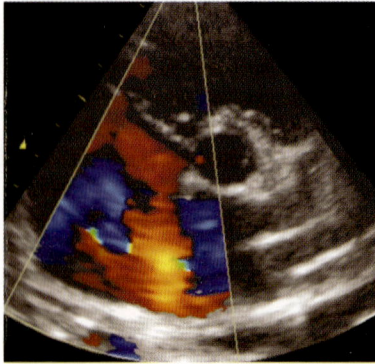

Figure 2.1: Color flow map extending from
left atrium to right atrium

chambers with dilated main pulmonary artery, prominent hila and pulmonary plethora. On ECHO, the right atrium and right ventricle were dilated and a signal drop-out was noticed in the interatrial septum. On colour Doppler, an abnormal flow map was observed extending across the area of echo drop-out, from the left atrium to the right atrium (Fig. 2.1). There were no abnormalities of the cardiac valves and the estimated pulmonary artery pressure was normal. Therefore, the definite diagnosis in this case is atrial septal defect (ASD).

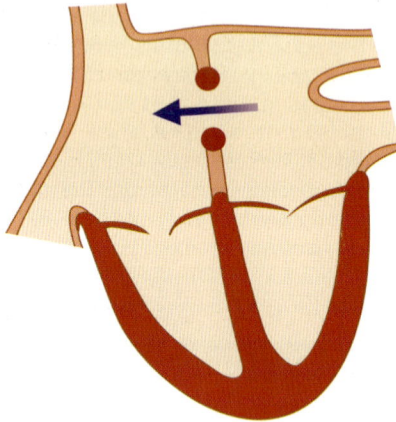

Figure 2.2: Atrial septal defect

In ASD, breach in the continuity of the interatrial septum creates a left-to-right shunt between the atria (Fig. 2.2). The septal defect occurs due to complexity of its embryological development. Most (75%) ASDs occur in the mid-portion of the septum, in the region of the foramen ovale and are termed as ostium secundum ASD. Some ASDs occur lower down the inter-atrial septum and are termed as ostium primum ASD (Fig. 2.3). Ostium primum ASDs are associated with cleft leaflets, regurgitation of the atrioventricular valves and are also known as endocardial cushion defect. An uncommon variety of ASD in the upper portion

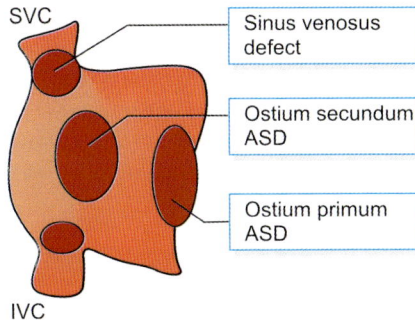

Figure 2.3: Various locations of atrial septal defect (ASD)
SVC: Superior vena cava; IVC: Inferior vena cava

Table 2.1: Types of atrial septal defect
• Ostium secundum ASD
• Ostium primum ASD
• Sinus venosus defect
• Vena caval defect

is sinus venosus defect, which is accompanied by anomalous pulmonary venous connections (Table 2.1). Inferior vena caval defects are very rare. An ASD may be associated with trisomy 21 (Down's syndrome) or abnormalities of the hand (Holt Oram syndrome).

The systolic murmur of ASD is due to increased flow across the pulmonary valve and not due to the shunt. The intensity of murmur does not correlate with the size of the ASD. However, a large ASD is associated with a diastolic flow murmur and a right-sided S_3, due to torrential flow across the tricuspid valve. An accompanying pansystolic murmur due to mitral and/or tricuspid regurgitation is a feature of ostium primum ASD. In ASD, the splitting of S_2 is wide and fixed. It is wide because of increased pulmonary ejection time, which delays the P_2.

Other reasons for wide splitting of S_2 are right bundle branch block or pulmonary stenosis (delayed P_2) and mitral regurgitation or ventricular septal defect (premature A_2). The splitting of S_2 is also wide in WPW syndrome Type A, in which there is pre-excitation of the left ventricle. The splitting of S_2 is fixed in ASD because the shunt equalizes atrial pressures throughout the respiratory cycle and there is no inspiratory augmentation of right ventricular filling.

On ECHO, since the signal from the interatrial septum is weak, false echo drop-out may be seen even in normal persons. The subcostal window may be a better option to diagnose an ASD but transesophageal echocardiography (TEE) provides excellent visualization particularly in endocardial cushion defects and sinus venosus ASD. Sometimes, contrast echo is needed to visualize the shunt using agitated saline, which contains air bubbles that cross over the septal defect.

ASD is the commonest congenital heart disease diagnosed in adulthood, with either absent or mild symptoms. It is 7 times more common in females than in males. Complications of ASD in adults are effort intolerance and pulmonary hypertension. Reversal of shunt and right heart failure are rare compared to ventricular septal defect. Atrial tachyarrhythmias including atrial fibrillation are common. Typically, sinus arrhythmia is never observed, because the shunt negates the effect of inspiration on venous return. Systemic thrombo-embolism can occur due to emboli from peripheral or pelvic veins, passing across the septal defect (paradoxical embolism).

MANAGEMENT ISSUES

Most ostium secundum atrial septal defects are amenable to percutaneous device closure. Large ASDs allow large volumes of left-to-right shunt and usually persent with exertional breathlessness and fatigue. They can lead to pulmonary hypertension and right heart failure, although reversal of shunt (right-to-left) is less common than in case of ventricular septal defect. Therefore, ASDs larger than 10 mm in size should ideally be closed before significant pulmonary hypertension develops.

Smaller ASDs with small volumes of shunt may become progressively more symptomatic as left ventricular compliance declines with age and the degree of shunting increases. Such ASDs that lead to right ventricular dilatation, should be closed during adulthood. Patients with ASD may develop paradoxical emboli which arise in the venous system and cross the septal defect to reach the systemic circulation. ASDs with history of thrombo-embolism should be closed, irrespective of their size (Table 2.2).

Table 2.2: Indications for surgical closure of ASD
• Large-sized ASD more than 10 mm in size with pulmonary to systemic flow ratio > 1.5:1
• Medium-sized ASD with dilated right ventricle without significant pulmonary hypertension
• Small-sized ASD without dilated right ventricle with history of systemic thrombo-embolism

Ostium primum atrial septal defects with atrioventricular valvular abnormalities and sinus venosus defects with anomalous pulmonary venous drainage are not amenable to percutaneous device closure because of their complexity. They require a definitive surgical procedure for their correction.

RECENT ADVANCES

Percutaneous deployment of a closure device for atrial septal defect has been standard practice for several decades. Transesophageal echocardiography (TEE) is widely used to guide the deployment. Recently, intracardiac ultrasound has been used to accurately assess the anatomy, for better selection and placement of the device. Vital anatomical information includes size of the defect, the rim around the defect and proximity to the mitral and tricuspid valves.

Fallot's Tetralogy

CASE PRESENTATION

A 14-year old girl was admitted to a tertiary-care hospital of a metropolitan city, with the complaint of progressive shortness of breath since 2 months, more so for the last 5 days. There was no history of fever, productive cough, chest pain or hemoptysis. The girl's mother also noticed an increase in the child's abdominal girth and swelling around both her ankles. The patient was born after a Caesarian section and was noticed to be cyanosed at birth. At the age of 3 years, the girl had undergone a surgical operation for congenital heart disease, in this very hospital. There was no history of repeated chest infection or childhood asthma, but the patient's growth milestones of early childhood were delayed.

On examination, the patient was slightly breathless at rest but was not distressed. The pulse rate was 84 beats/min., with a BP of 96/66 mm Hg. There was cyanosis over the tongue and lips and the finger-tips and toes were clubbed. Pitting ankle edema was present and the neck veins were engorged. Per abdomen findings were a 5 cm hepatomegaly with mild ascites. The breath sounds were vesicular in character without any rhonchi or crepts. On precordial examination, the apex beat was normal in location with a left parasternal heave. Auscultation revealed a normal S_1 and S_2 with an early-diastolic murmur over the pulmonary area and a soft pansystolic murmur over the lower left parasternal area.

CLINICAL DISCUSSION

From the history and physical examination, this young girl had congenital cyanotic heart disease that was operated upon during her early childhood. At present she was in right heart failure with pulmonary and tricuspid valve regurgitation and had right ventricular enlargement. Right ventricular enlargement is associated with a palpable left parasternal heave. Common causes of right ventricular enlargement are pulmonary valve stenosis and pulmonary arterial hypertension. The commonest cause of pulmonary regurgitation is pulmonary hypertension, but it can also follow a surgical procedure on the pulmonary valve. Rare causes of pulmonary regurgitation are subvalvular pulmonary stenosis and carcinoid syndrome (Table 3.1). Functional tricuspid regurgitation (dilated annulus) is a consequence of right ventricular dilatation due to any cause. Tricuspid regurgitation is associated with raised JVP with prominent v waves and rapid

Table 3.1: Causes of pulmonary regurgitation
• Primary: Carcinoid syndrome
• Congenital: Subvalvular stenosis
• Iatrogenic: Pulmonary valvotomy
• Secondary: Pulmonary hypertension

y descent. An enlarged pulsatile liver with a pansystolic murmur over the lower left parasternal area are also observed.

ECG showed sinus rhythm with tall R waves in right precordial leads and T wave inversion, suggestive of right ventricular hypertrophy with strain (Fig. 3.1). P. pulmonale and right axis deviation of the QRS were also seen. X-ray chest findings were increased cardio-thoracic ratio with reduced pulmonary vascular markings and a right-sided aortic arch. On ECHO, the left ventricle was normal in size with an ejection fraction of 55% but the right ventricle was significantly dilated. The mitral and aortic valves were normal in structure but there was moderate pulmonary regurgitation and significant tricuspid regurgitation.

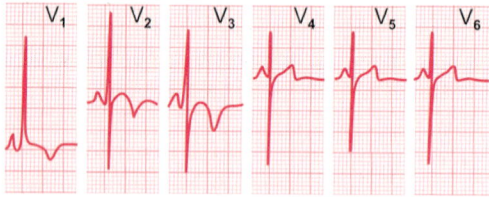

Figure 3.1: ECG showing tall R waves in leads V_1 to V_3.

This patient was operated upon for a cardiac defect, when she was 3 years old. The most common congenital cyanotic heart disease that is associated with survival until adolescence and sometimes even into adulthood is tetralogy of Fallot. Therefore, in all probability, this patient was operated upon for Fallot's tetralogy and had now developed pulmonary regurgitation (Fig. 3.2), as a complication of the surgical procedure on the pulmonary valve. The right ventricular enlargement that ensued, led to secondary tricuspid regurgitation because of annular dilatation.

Tetralogy of Fallot is the most common congenital cyanotic heart disease that survives into adolescence. It is associated with a right-to-left shunt since birth unlike isolated septal defects which are left-to-right shunts and undergo reversal only after the development of pulmonary hypertension. The four components (Fig. 3.3) of Fallot's tetralogy are:
- Pulmonary stenosis (PS)
- Overriding of aorta (OA)
- Ventricular septal defect (VSD)
- Right ventricular hypertrophy (RVH)

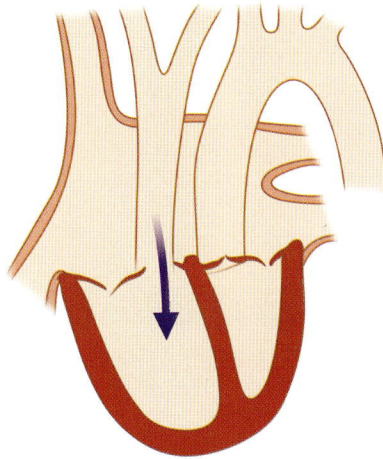

Figure 3.2: Pulmonary regurgitation

The primary developmental abnormality is of the pulmonary subvalvular or infundibular area leading to pulmonary stenosis (PS) and right ventricular outflow tract (RVOT) obstruction. Rarely, the pulmonary valve is absent (pulmonary atresia). The ventricular septal defect (VSD) is membranous in location. The aorta is displaced rightward and overrides the septum, the overriding aorta (OA). Therefore, the septum is not in line with the anterior aortic wall but with the aortic valve closure point. The right ventricular hypertrophy (RVH) is secondary to RVOT obstruction. Rarely, an atrial septal defect (ASD) may be associated, in which case the constellation is designated as pentalogy of Fallot.

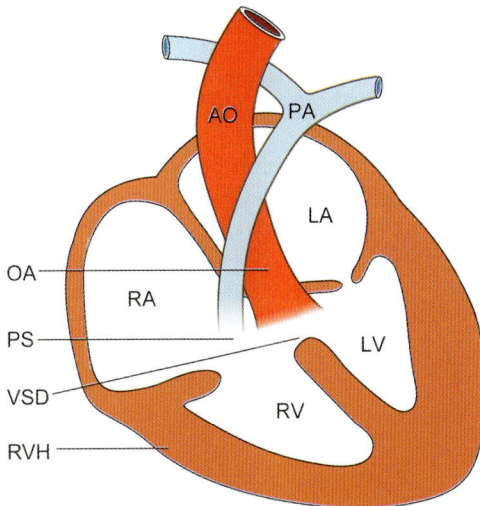

Figure 3.3: The four components of Fallot's tetralogy. AO: Aorta; OA: Overriding aorta; RA: Right atrium; LA: Left atrium; RV: Right ventricle; LV: Left ventricle PS: Pulmonary stenosis; PA: Pulmonary artery; VSD: Ventricular septal defect; RVH: Right ventricular hypertrophy

In a typical unrepaired case of Fallot's tetralogy, auscultatory findings are a loud, single S_2 and a parasternal systolic murmur. The S_2 is single because the P_2 is muffled and the A_2 is loud because the aorta is anteriorly placed. The systolic murmur originates from the subvalvular pulmonary stenosis and not from the ventricular septal defect. The classical clinical features of Fallot's tetralogy are central cyanosis, finger clubbing, anoxic spells, growth retardation and exercise intolerance. Congestive heart failure is rare because the septal defect balances the right and left ventricular pressures. If left unrepaired, catastrophic complications in adolescence are arterial thrombo-embolism and cerebral abscess.

MANAGEMENT ISSUES

Until the 1970s and even early-1980s, surgical interventions in very early childhood were largely palliative. These shunt procedures were performed to bypass the RVOT obstruction and to enhance pulmonary blood flow. These shunts were Blalock-Taussig shunt (subclavian artery to pulmonary artery) and Waterston shunt (ascending aorta to right pulmonary artery). However, even after these procedures, patients remained symptomatic and complications occurred unabated. Nowadays, total surgical correction is undertaken to close the shunt and to enhance pulmonary blood flow. This includes patch closure of the VSD with pulmonary subvalvular muscle resection and valvotomy.

Cardiac surgeons are increasingly encountering complications of prior surgical correction, as these children survive into their teens. Complications after surgery include residual shunt, residual stenosis or, post-valvotomy pulmonary regurgitation and right ventricular enlargement as in our case. Pulmonary valve replacement with tricuspid annular repair would be the best course of action in this case.

RECENT ADVANCES

Prior cardiac surgery often distorts the anatomy of the heart to an extent that the information obtained from transthoracic echocardiography is generally skewed and inconclusive. Modern cardiac imaging techniques of computed tomography (CT) and magnetic resonance imaging (MRI) are particularly useful to evaluate postoperative patients.

Percutaneous techniques are currently being evaluated in the management of Fallot's tetralogy. Pulmonary balloon angioplasty and artificial valve deployment by non-surgical intervention have been recently described.

C A S E

4

Ebstein's Anomaly

CASE PRESENTATION

A 26-year old married woman visited a cardiologist's chamber, with the complaint of occasional fluttering sensation in the chest of 2 years duration. The episodes of palpitation were associated with some light-headedness, but she had never fainted. Her palpitation was at times related to some emotional upset or undue physical exercise, but there was no history of exertional fatigue, chest pain or breathlessness. There was also no history of tremor of the hands or weight loss. Her childhood had been uneventful with normal growth milestones and there was no history of cyanotic spells during sports activities. She also denied having had recurrent sore-throat, joint pains or any prolonged febrile illness during her school days.

On examination, the patient was comfortable, relaxed and not dyspneic. There was no tremor of the fingers, visible goiter or eye-signs of Grave's disease. The JVP was raised 5 cm above the angle of Louis and showed large v waves with a prominent y descent. The pulse was regular, fair in volume, at a rate of 84 beats/min. and the BP was 130/80 mm Hg. On examining the abdomen, there were visible epigastric pulsations, with the liver edge 6 cm below the right costal margin and pulsatile; no ascites was demonstrable. The apex beat was normal in nature and location but a left parasternal heave was palpated. The S_1 and S_2 were both split with wide splitting of S_2 appreciated during inspiration. No S_3 or S_4 gallop sound was heard. A pansystolic murmur was audible at the lower end of the left sternal edge. Breathing was vesicular and no rhonchi or crepts were heard over the lung fields.

CLINICAL DISCUSSION

From the history and physical examination, this patient had paroxysmal tachycardia with clinical signs of tricuspid valve regurgitation. ECG showed tall P waves (P. pulmonale) with normal P-R interval and right bundle branch block (RBBB). X-ray chest finding was an enlarged cardiac silhouette, more so towards the right of the midline. ECHO revealed normal sized left ventricle with normal ejection fraction. The mitral and aortic valves were normal and the left atrium was not dilated. There was no echo drop-out in the region of either septum. However, the right atrium was markedly enlarged and the right ventricle was dilated as well as hyperkinetic. The tricuspid valve was displaced downwards into the right ventricle, with distal attachment of the septal tricuspid leaflet which showed exaggerated excursion. On colour flow mapping, a regurgitant jet was seen in the right atrium. These findings are consistent with the diagnosis of Ebstein's anomaly.

In a young woman, history of episodic palpitation raises several clinical possibilities. Anxiety neurosis, panic attacks and paroxysmal supraventricular tachycardia are usual causes but in these, the heart is structurally normal. Perimenopausal symptoms in women include palpitation but our patient was young. Thyrotoxicosis is a possibility but our patient had no goiter, tremor or eye-signs of Grave's disease. Pre-excitation syndrome (WPW syndrome) may be responsible for paroxysmal tachyarrhythmia but the ECG did not show short P-R interval or delta waves on the QRS complex. Mitral valve prolapse (MVP) and atrial septal defect (ASD) are structural cardiac abnormalities that are responsible for tachyarrhythmias. However, in our case the mitral valve was normal and there was no septal defect.

Ebstein's anomaly is an uncommon congenital acyanotic heart disease characterized by abnormal tricuspid valve architecture, tricuspid regurgitation and association with paroxysmal supraventricular tachyarrhythmias. The physical examination of the patient and interpretation of simple cardiac investigations is a good exercise in bed-side clinical cardiology. A raised JVP with large v waves and prominent y descent are characteristic of tricuspid regurgitation into the right atrium (Fig. 4.1). So is an enlarged and pulsatile liver on abdominal examination. A sustained left parasternal heave is indicative of right ventricular volume overload.

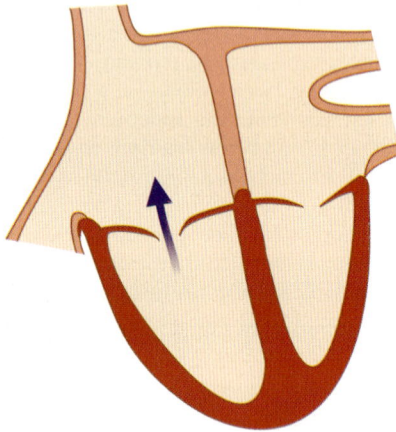

Figure 4.1: Tricuspid regurgitation

The S_1 is split because of delayed tricuspid valve closure (T_1) due to right bundle branch block (RBBB) as well as the wide excursion of the septal tricuspid leaflet. The S_2 is widely split due to delayed pulmonary closure (P_2) because of the RBBB. Sometimes, the S_2 is single because of soft P_2 due to low pulmonary ejection volume. Rarely, the S_2 is paradoxically split because of pre-excitation of the right ventricle caused by WPW syndrome Type B. The pansystolic murmur of tricuspid regurgitation is best audible over the lower left parasternal area and does not radiate towards the axilla or the base of the heart. Like all right-sided murmurs, it

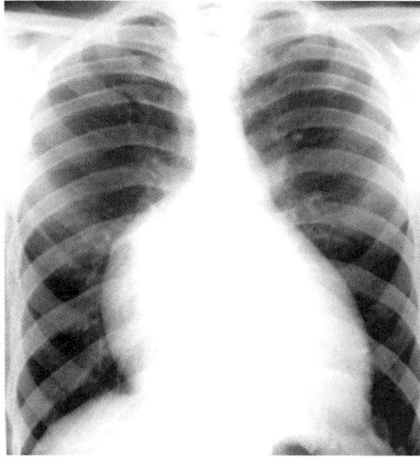

Figure 4.2: X-ray showing cardiomegaly due
to enlargement of right atrium

increases in intensity during inspiration, provided the right ventricular function
is normal.

In sinus rhythm, the ECG shows tall P waves (P. pulmonale) due to right atrial
enlargement and wide QRS complexes due to right bundle branch block (RBBB).
Sometimes, wide QRS complexes are due to WPW syndrome, in which case there
is a short P-R interval (pre-excitation). At times, the rhythm is atrial fibrillation.
On X-ray chest, the cardiac silhouette is enlarged towards the right of the midline,
due to the large right atrium (Fig. 4.2). Superficially, this resembles a pericardial
effusion. The differentiating feature is that the right lower portion of the cardiac
silhouette curves inwards towards the center of the chest and not outwards, as it
would in case of pericardial effusion.

On ECHO apical view, there is downward displacement of the tricuspid
valve into the body of the right ventricle, towards the apex. The septal tricuspid

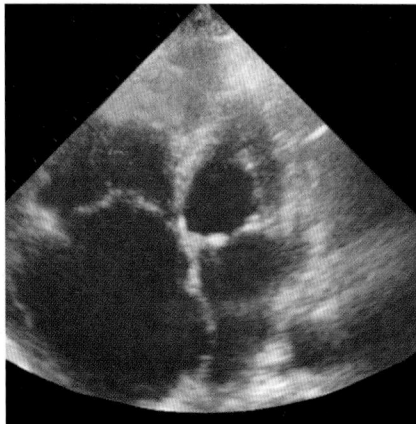

Figure 4.3: ECHO showing enlarged right atrium
with displaced tricuspid valve

leaflet is attached to the IV septum, 10 mm or more distal to the anterior mitral leaflet. The tricuspid leaflet is large and shows wide excursion, often with a whip-like motion. The right ventricle is dilated and hyperkinetic due to volume overload. The right atrium is enlarged because of tricuspid regurgitation as well as due to "atrialization" of the upper portion of the right ventricle (Fig. 4.3). On long-axis view, because of downward displacement of the tricuspid valve, there is simultaneous recording of the mitral and tricuspid valves (MV and TV). On short-axis view, the tricuspid valve is shifted clockwise, from the normal 9 0'clock position to the 11 0'clock position.

The commonest reason for tricuspid regurgitation is dilatation of the tricuspid valve annulus secondary to right ventricular dilatation. Reason for annular dilatation is usually pulmonary hypertension due to congenital left-to-right shunt, rheumatic mitral valve disease or chronic cor pulmonale. Sometimes, dilated cardiomyopathy causes annular dilatation (Table 4.1). Primary tricuspid valvular regurgitation has several causes except coronary artery disease and systemic hypertension, the commonest forms of heart disease. Usual causes of tricuspid valve regurgitation are tricuspid leaflet prolapse, Ebstein's anomaly, rheumatic heart disease, carcinoid syndrome and right-sided endocarditis. Uncommon causes include endocardial cushion defects, endomyocardial fibrosis and connective tissue disorders.

Table 4.1: Causes of tricuspid regurgitation
Valvular regurgitation
• Tricuspid valve prolapse
• Right-sided endocarditis
• Ebstein's anomaly
• Carcinoid syndrome
• Endocardial cushion defect
• Endomyocardial fibrosis
• Connective tissue disease
Annular dilatation
• Pulmonary hypertension
• Pulmonary regurgitation
• Dilated cardiomyopathy

MANAGEMENT ISSUES

The management of Ebstein's anomaly includes the treatment of supraventricular tachyarrhythmias and the control of tricuspid regurgitation. Drugs that block the atrioventricular (AV) node to reduce the heart rate, such as betablockers and verapamil, are the agents of choice. In the presence of WPW syndrome, amiodarone is preferable. Digoxin may be used to treat atrial fibrillation in which case, an anticoagulant is also prescribed to reduce the risk of thrombo-embolism. If the tachyarrhythmias are refractory to drug treatment or an accessory bypass tract is present, radiofrequency ablation can be offered. In the presence of moderate to severe tricuspid regurgitation, valve repair with restrictive annuloplasty or even valve replacement may be considered.

5

Patent Ductus Arteriosus

CASE PRESENTATION

A 6-year old boy was taken to the pediatrician by his mother, for treatment of fever with coryza and cough. While auscultating the chest of the child, the pediatrician incidentally heard a loud murmur over the upper precordium. Although the child had been taken to several doctors in the past for consultation and vaccination, nobody had noticed the murmur. The boy was born after normal vaginal delivery, without any intervention and was not cyanosed at birth. His mother had experienced no difficulty in nursing him. The boy's growth milestones of early childhood were not delayed.

On examination, the child was irritable because of his respiratory catarrhe but not tachypneic. He was febrile but not anemic or icteric and there was no cyanosis or clubbing of the fingers or toes. The extremities were warm but not sweaty and his radial pulse was bounding in nature at a rate of 110 beats/min. The thyroid gland was not enlarged and there was no sign of congestive heart failure. The BP over the right arm in the supine position was 160/60 mm Hg and similar in the left arm. The child's mother was quite sure that his blood pressure had never been checked earlier.

On examination of the precordium, the apex beat was hyperkinetic but there was no palpable parasternal heave. The loud murmur over the precordium was wide-spread but maximally audible in the 2nd left intercostal space, just below the middle of the left clavicle. On careful auscultation, the murmur was pansystolic but extended upto and through S_2, well into diastole. No S_3 or S_4 sound could be appreciated because of the long murmur. The lung fields were clear on auscultation without any rhonchi or crepitations.

CLINICAL DISCUSSION

From the history and physical examination, this boy had a bounding pulse and an incidentally detected systolo-diastolic murmur. A good volume radial pulse, which can be appreciated even with the arm elevated above the head, is known as collapsing pulse. A collapsing pulse is indicative of a wide pulse pressure. Causes of a wide pulse pressure are:

- Severe anemia
- Thyrotoxicosis
- Paget's disease
- Beri-beri disease
- Aortic regurgitation

- Arterio-venous fistula
- Patent ductus arteriosus.

A long murmur that extends throughout systole and crosses S_2 to spill over into diastole, is known as a continuous murmur. Causes of a continuous murmur are as follows:

- Venous hum
- Mammary souffle
- Coarctation of aorta
- Patent ductus arteriosus
- Aortopulmonary window
- Coronary arterio-venous fistula
- Ruptured aneurysm sinus of Valsalva

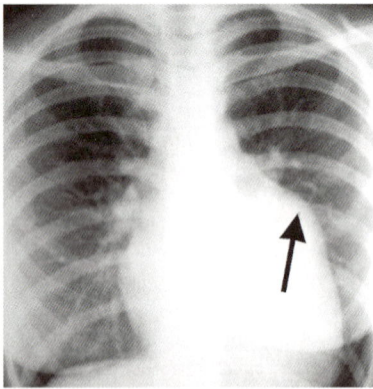

Figure 5.1: X-ray showing cardiomegaly with prominent pulmonary artery

ECG of the patient showed tall R waves in left precordial leads and deep S waves in right precordial leads. X-ray chest findings were cardiomegaly with left ventricular contour and a prominent main pulmonary artery with pulmonary plethora (Fig. 5.1). On ECHO, the left ventricle was dilated with normal systolic function. The left atrium was also dilated and all cardiac valves were structurally normal. On colour flow mapping, there was a retrograde mosaic jet extending from the left pulmonary artery to the dilated main pulmonary artery (Fig. 5.2).

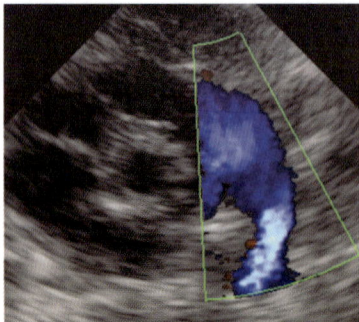

Figure 5.2: ECHO showing retrograde jet from left branch to main pulmonary artery

On pulsed-wave Doppler, with the sample volume moving distally from the right ventricular outflow tract and across the pulmonary valve, increased velocity was detected in the pulmonary artery. The estimated pulmonary artery pressure was normal. Therefore, the definite diagnosis in this case is patent ductus arteriosus.

The ductus arteriosus is a channel that connects the descending aorta distal to the origin of left subclavian artery, to the left pulmonary artery just distal to the bifurcation of main pulmonary artery. The ductus remains open during intrauterine life and closes soon after birth when its purpose is fulfilled. When the ductus fails to close physiologically within 24 hours after birth and anatomically within a week, it provides a communication between the aortic and pulmonary circulations. Flow from the aorta (at higher pressure) to the pulmonary artery (at lower pressure) creates a left-to-right shunt across the PDA (Fig. 5.3). Persistence of the ductus is sometimes associated with maternal rubella syndrome and premature delivery.

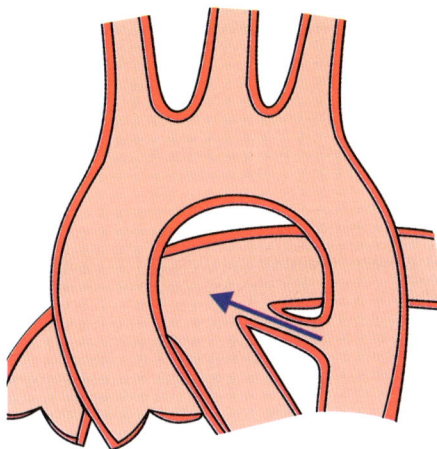

Figure 5.3: Patent ductus arteriosus

The continuous murmur of PDA is classically described as a "machinery" murmur and is referred to as Gibson's murmur. It is maximally audible below the middle of the left clavicle, just before and just after the S_2. The continuous murmur may be accompanied by a mid-diastolic murmur over the mitral area, due to torrential flow across the mitral valve. There may also be reverse splitting of S_2, due to delayed closure of the aortic valve. When pulmonary hypertension develops, the murmur of PDA is confined to systole.

As already mentioned, there are several causes of a continuous murmur. In aorto-pulmonary window, there is a proximal communication between the aorta and the pulmonary artery. Although the murmur of aortic coarctation is typically systolic, in tight stenosis the murmur may extend into diastole. Venous hum is a low-pitched continuous murmur which is loudest over the supraclavicular fossa, but sometimes also heard over the precordium. It is accentuated by looking over the shoulder while sitting and abolished by compression of the jugular vein.

A mammary soufflé is heard widely over the precordium in pregnant women. It is better appreciated while lying down and during systole. Coronary fistula and ruptured aneurysm of sinus of Valsalva are rare arterio-venous communications that can also produce a continuous murmur.

Ventricular septal defect (VSD) produces a pansystolic murmur while aortic regurgitation causes an early diastolic murmur. When the two are associated as in perimembranous VSD, the murmur is systolo-diastolic. A similar systolo-diastolic murmur occurs when an atrial septal defect (ASD) is associated with mitral stenosis, the Lutembacher syndrome. In contrast to a continuous murmur, the two components of a systolo-diastolic murmur have a different character.

PDA is the commonest cause of cardiomegaly and heart failure in infancy and childhood. Conversely, heart failure is the commonest cause of morbidity and mortality in PDA, at any age. Causes of heart failure in childhood are:

- Coarctation of aorta
- Patent ductus arteriosus
- Congenital cardiomyopathy
- Anomalous left coronary artery arising from pulmonary artery (ALCAPA).

When pulmonary hypertension develops in PDA, reversal of the shunt from pulmonary artery to aorta may occur. In that case, the continuous murmur gets shorter and quieter. The toes get more cyanosed and clubbed than the fingers. The reason for this differential cyanosis is that the ductus is distal to the left subclavian artery and predominantly the lower limbs get deoxygenated blood. Other complication of PDA are endarteritis, aneurysm formation and rarely rupture of the ductus.

MANAGEMENT ISSUES

Percutaneous device closure of patent ductus arteriosus was one of the earliest non-surgical interventions in cardiology. All PDAs of significant size and shunt should be ligated, except in ductus dependent complex congenital cyanotic heart diseases of infancy.

Mitral Valve Diseases

Mitral
Stenosis

CASE PRESENTATION

A 23-year old woman of low socio-economic status came to a general hospital with shortness of breath, fatigue and palpitations since 2 years and fever with productive cough for the last 1 week. She denied any chest pain, wheezing or hemoptysis. At the age of 12, she had a prolonged febrile illness with joint pains and ever since, she had been receiving monthly injections of penicillin.

On examination she was tachypneic with pallor but there was no cyanosis or icterus. Pulse rate was 96 beats/min. regular, with a BP of 100/70 mm Hg. Her temperature was 100^0 F. The JVP was not raised, thyroid gland was not enlarged and there were no palpable lymph nodes. There was no evidence of pharyngo-tonsillitis, swollen joints or petechial spots over the skin, eyes or finger-tips. The apex beat was tapping in nature with a left parasternal heave. The S_1 was loud and the P_2 was also accentuated. A low-pitched mid-diastolic rumbling murmur was heard over the cardiac apex. The murmur was preceded by an opening snap and accentuated just before systole. There were scattered rhonchi and crepts over the lung fields.

CLINICAL DISCUSSION

From the history and physical examination, this young woman in all probability had rheumatic heart disease with mitral valve stenosis (Fig. 6.1). The S_1 is loud

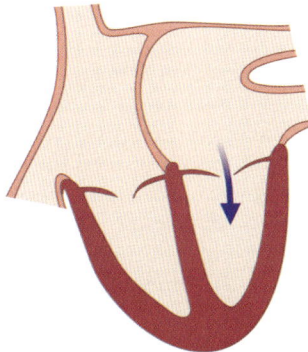

Figure 6.1: Mitral valve stenosis

since the mitral valve leaflets are distant from each other at the end of diastole and snap together loudly. Other reasons for a loud S_1 are sinus tachycardia and a short P-R interval, where the diastole is short. The mid-diastolic murmur of mitral stenosis (MS) is best heard with the patient in the left lateral decubitus position, using the stethoscope bell.

The length of the murmur correlates with the severity of stenosis. The murmur undergoes presystolic accentuation due to atrial contribution to ventricular filling. In mild MS, the murmur may be only presystolic. If MS is associated with atrial fibrillation the S_1 is variable in intensity due to variable duration of diastole. Also, presystolic accentuation is lost due to lack of atrial contribution to ventricular filling. Presystolic accentuation is also absent in a calcified valve and after commissurotomy. Severe mitral stenosis may be silent due to low cardiac output and the fact that the right ventricle underlies most of the precordium because of clockwise cardiac rotation.

The opening snap heralds the onset of ventricular diastolic filling and the end of isovolumic relaxation. It indicates pliability of the valve, suitability for valvotomy and is absent in a heavily calcified valve or after commissurotomy. An early opening snap after A_2 (short 2A-OS interval), indicates higher left atrial pressure and more severe MS. Besides mitral stenosis, other reasons for a mid-diastolic murmur are acute rheumatic valvulitis (Carey-Coomb murmur), aortic regurgitation (Austin-Flint murmur), left atrial myxoma (prolapse into mitral orifice) and left-to-right shunt (increased transmitral inflow).

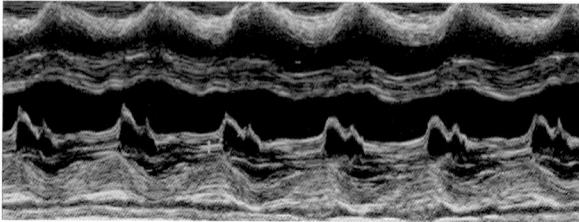

Figure 6.2: M-mode ECHO showing reduced excursion of AML with paradoxical motion of PML

ECG showed sinus rhythm, P mitrale, right ventricular hypertrophy with a rightward QRS axis. X-ray chest findings were straightening of the left heart border with pulmonary congestion. On M-mode ECHO, excursion of the anterior leaflet was reduced with paradoxical excursion of the posterior leaflet (Fig. 6.2). On 2-D ECHO, the left atrium and right ventricle were dilated. The mitral valve leaflets were thickened with limited excursion and restricted valve opening. The anterior mitral leaflet showed diastolic doming (Fig. 6.3). There was no abnormality of the aortic valve and the estimated pulmonary artery pressure was elevated.

The severity of mitral stenosis can be gauged and classified, according to several calculated indices from echocardiography. These are the pressure gradient across the valve (PG), the time taken for the PG to fall to half (P½t; pressure half-time), the pulmonary artery pressure (PAP) estimated from the peak tricuspid velocity (TR Vmax) and the mitral valve area (MVA) calculated by planimetry (Table 6.1). However, there are some fallacies associated with these

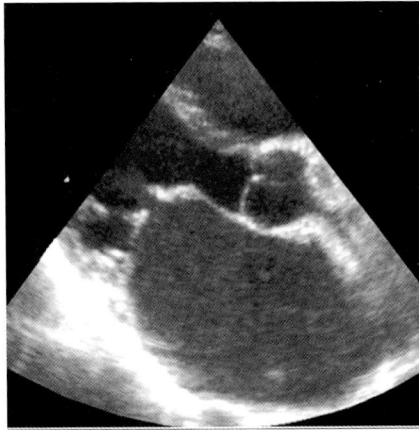

Figure 6.3: 2-D ECHO showing restricted opening with diastolic doming and dilated left atrium

Table 6.1: Assessment of the severity of mitral stenosis			
	Mild	Moderate	Severe
PG (mm Hg)	< 5	5-10	>10
P½ t (msec)	<150	150-220	>220
TRV$_{max}$ (m/sec)	<2.7	2.7-3.0	>3.0
PAP (mm Hg)	<30	30-50	>50
MVA (cm^2)	>1.5	1.0-1.5	<1.0

calculations. The peak velocity and pressure gradient depend on the heart rate and stroke volume. Measurement of mitral valve area may be fallacious due to heavily calcified leaflets, subvalvular pathology and prior commissurotomy.

Rheumatic heart disease is the predominant cause of mitral stenosis. 80% of cases are women in the 2nd or 3rd decade of life, from the developing countries. Rare causes are congenital MS (parachute valve), mucopolysaccharidosis (Hurler's syndrome), severe annular calcification and connective tissue disorders (Table 6.2). Complications of MS are pulmonary congestion, respiratory infections, hemoptysis, right heart failure and systemic thrombo-embolism due to atrial fibrillation associated with left atrial thrombus.

Table 6.2: Causes of mitral stenosis
• Rheumatic heart disease (commonest)
• Congenital parachute valve
• Mitral annular calcification
• Connective tissue disorder
• Hurler's mucopolysaccharidosis

PERTINENT INVESTIGATIONS

Since rheumatic heart disease is the predominant cause of mitral stenosis, all patients who are febrile should be investigated for rheumatic fever, infective endocarditis and respiratory tract infection. Relevant investigations are Hb, TLC, DLC, ESR, urine R/E, CRP value and ASLO titre. Throat-swab culture for beta-hemolytic Streptococcus and bacterial blood cultures may be included.

Transthoracic ECHO is central to the diagnosis and assessment of mitral stenosis. Besides determining the severity of MS, it can assess left atrial size, left ventricular function and estimate pulmonary artery pressure. Transesophageal echocardiography (TEE) allows better assessment of the subvalvular and commissural architecture and improves the detection of a left atrial thrombus.

MANAGEMENT ISSUES

All patients of mitral stenosis should be offered penicillin prophylaxis against rheumatic fever, until they attain the age of 40 years. A broad-spectrum antimicrobial agent should be administered prior to any invasive dental or surgical procedure, to guard against infective endocarditis. Diuretics reduce pulmonary congestion, especially in patients with associated mitral or aortic regurgitation. Rate control with digoxin, beta-blocker or verapamil improves left ventricular diastolic filling, in patients who are in sinus rhythm and controls the ventricular response, in whom the rhythm is atrial fibrillation. Since atrial fibrillation in patients with mitral stenosis is associated with a high risk of thrombo-embolism, these patients should also be on a long-term oral anticoagulant agent like warfarin.

Percutaneous balloon mitral valvuloplasty (BMV) is the procedure of choice in symptomatic severe mitral stenosis, provided a transesophageal echocardiography (TEE) does not reveal subvalvular fusion, commissural calcification, atrial thrombus or more than mild MR (Table 6.3). Recurrence of symptoms after valvotomy is more often due to induced mitral regurgitation rather than restenosis. If valvotomy cannot be performed because of the aforementioned reasons, mitral valve replacement (MVR) is undertaken. During MVR, if atrial fibrillation is present, left atrial radiofrequency ablation (RFA) and appendage ligation are also performed.

Table 6.3: Indications for valvotomy in MS

The absence of concomitant:
- Subvalvular fusion
- Left atrial thrombus
- Immobility of leaflets
- Commissural calcification
- Moderate/severe regurgitation

RECENT ADVANCES

Although transesophageal echocardiography (TEE) has vastly improved acquisition of detailed information over the transthoracic approach, multi-slice computed tomography (CT) is being increasingly used to accurately assess the area and the precise nature of the mitral valve.

7

Mitral Regurgitation

CASE PRESENTATION

A 46-year old woman of stocky built, was asked to see a cardiologist by her family doctor. She complained of exertional shortness of breath and had a cardiac murmur. She was a known case of hypertension, adequately controlled by medication. Her breathlessness had been felt since the last 4 months but had significantly worsened over the preceding 2 weeks. There was no history of exertional chest pain or of palpitation and fainting. She did not smoke or consume alcohol but she seldom exercised and did not follow the diet-plan suggested by her physician.

On examination, she was overweight without any clinical signs of cortisol excess or hypothyroidism. The pulse was regular, good in volume at a rate of 92 beats/min. The BP was 136/88 mm Hg in the right arm. There was no sign of heart failure. The apex beat was hyperdynamic, ill-sustained heaving in nature and displaced towards the left axilla. The S_1 was soft. A_2 was loud and a soft S_3 was audible in early diastole. A soft blowing pansystolic murmur was audible over the mitral area, that radiated towards the axilla. Also, a short diastolic rumble was heard over the cardiac apex. Few basilar rales were auscultated over the lower lung fields.

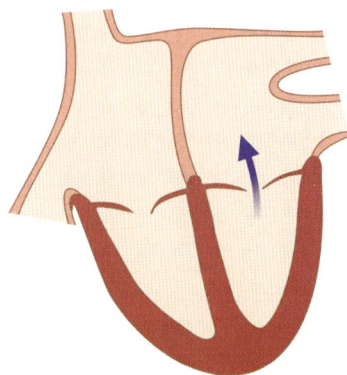

Figure 7.1: Mitral regurgitation

CLINICAL DISCUSSION

From the history and physical examination, this woman had mitral regurgitation (Fig. 7.1) with possibly associated mitral stenosis and evidence of left ventricular dilatation. The S$_1$ was soft since the mitral leaflets are close to each other at the end of diastole and snap together softly. The A$_2$ was loud due to associated systemic hypertension. The displacement of the apex beat and audible S$_3$ sound are indicative of left ventricular diastolic overload. The S$_3$ is a low-pitched sound that follows the A$_2$. It indicates abrupt halting of left ventricular filling. Physiological S$_3$ is appreciated in mitral regurgitation, left-to-right shunt and high cardiac output states. Pathological S$_3$ is audible in aortic regurgitation and left ventricular systolic dysfunction.

The pansystolic murmur of mitral regurgitation typically radiates to the left axilla (and sometimes even to the left scapula), if the anterior mitral leaflet is diseased. It radiates to the base of the heart, if the posterior mitral leaflet is involved. This differentiates it from the pansystolic murmur of tricuspid regurgitation or a ventricular septal defect. The accompanying diastolic rumble does not necessarily indicate concomitant mitral stenosis and is due to torrential flow across the valve, which is the sum of normal atrial blood volume and the regurgitant volume. It is worth mentioning that the murmur of acute or severe MR is not pansystolic but early systolic, because less turbulence is generated by the large valve orifice. Moreover, the rapid rise of left atrial pressure impedes regurgitation during later systole. The murmur of mitral annular calcification is also typically early systolic.

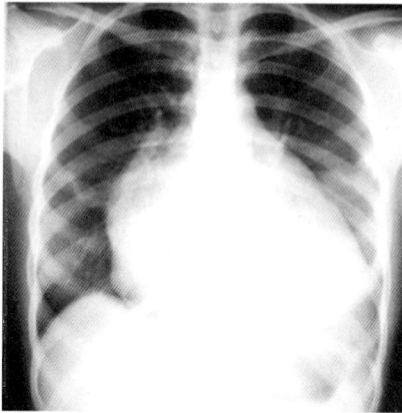

Figure 7.2: X-ray showing cardiac enlargement straightening of left heart border

ECG of the patient showed tall R waves in left precordial leads with upright T waves, indicating left ventricular diastolic overload. X-ray chest findings were moderate cardiomegaly, pulmonary congestion and straightening of the left heart border (Fig. 7.2). The "4-bump" left heart border is due to a large left atrial appendage, which is damaged during acute carditis and bulges due to high left atrial pressure in rheumatic mitral regurgitation (MR). On ECHO, the left ventricle was dilated and hyperkinetic with an ejection fraction of 55% and left atrial enlargement. Importantly, in functional MR due to annular dilatation secondary to cardiomyopathy, there is global hypokinesia of the left ventricle or a regional wall motion abnormality. In acute MR due to ruptured chordae tendinae, there is minimal left ventricular dilatation. The mitral valve leaflets were thickened and fibrotic indicating rheumatic MR. Other potential abnormalities of the mitral valve in case of MR are mitral leaflet redundancy and prolapse, flail leaflet, annular calcification or vegetations in case of endocarditis.

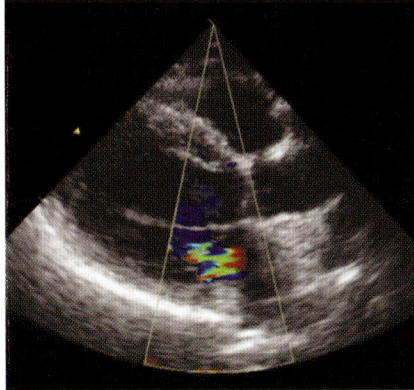

Figure 7.3: ECHO showing a color-flow map
in the left atrium

On colour flow mapping, a regurgitant jet was seen entering the left atrium (Fig. 7.3). The volume of MR (ml/beat), the MR jet area (cm^2) and the percentage of left atrial area (%) filled by the jet are used to gauge the severity of MR (Table 7.1). However, there are some fallacies associated with these calculations. The spatial profile of the MR jet does not truly reflect the regurgitant volume. It depends upon the shape of the valve orifice, the angle of the jet, left ventricular filling pressure and the size of the left atrium. The MR jet may be "eccentric" or "off-centre" in case of leaflet prolapse, papillary muscle rupture and paraprosthetic leak.

Table 7.1: Assessment of the severity of mitral regurgitation			
	Mild	**Moderate**	**Severe**
MR jet area (cm^2)	<4	4-8	>8
Percent of LA area (%)	<25	25-50	>50
MR Volume (ml/beat)	<30	30-59	>60
LV dysfunction	**Mild-to-moderate**		**Severe**
Ejection fraction (%)	30-60		<30
LV diameter (mm)	40-55		>55

There are several causes of mitral regurgitation (MR). Usual causes of primary MR are rheumatic heart disease, mitral leaflet prolapse, papillary muscle dysfunction, infective endocarditis and mitral annular calcification. Uncommon causs include congenital endocardial cushion defects, endomyocardial fibrosis

Table 7.2: Causes of mitral regurgitation
Chronic MR
• Mitral valve prolapse
• Dilated cardiomyopathy
• Endomyocardial fibrosis
• Rheumatic heart disease
• Mitral annular calcification
• Connective tissue disorder
• Papillary muscle dysfunction
Acute MR
• Acute myocardial infarction
• Infective endocarditis
• Blunt chest trauma.

and connective tissue disorders. Occasionally, secondary MR is due to mitral annular dilatation, as a result of dilated or ischemic cardiomyopathy. Acute MR can result from rupture of papillary muscle or chordae tendinae in case of myocardial infarction, infective endocarditis or after blunt trauma to the chest (Table 7.2).

MANAGEMENT ISSUES

Patients of rheumatic MR below the age of 40 should receive penicillin prophylaxis to protect them from acute rheumatic fever. Those undergoing a dental or surgical procedure, need antibiotic prophylaxis against infective endocarditis. Vasodilators such as ACE inhibitors or ARBs combined with a diuretic relieve pulmonary congestion, especially if systemic hypertension is present. Digoxin and an anticoagulant are used if there is concomitant atrial fibrillation. Secondary MR is reduced by lowering preload and afterload, which decrease the diameter of the mitral annulus.

Surgical operations for MR are mitral valve repair and valve replacement. Repair of the valve or annuloplasty is preferable if the valvular anatomy is suitable, since it preserves left ventricular geometry and spares the patient from the problems of anticoagulation. Replacement of the valve is indicated if the valvular anatomy is severely distorted.

RECENT ADVANCES

Mitral regurgitation in the context of ischemic heart disease is a clinical challenge. The MR is not due to an intrinsic valvular abnormality, but the result of ventricular dilatation with annular enlargement, papillary muscle dysfunction and dysfunctional ventricular remodeling with increased sphericity. These patients can be offered restrictive annuloplasty, which involves insertion of an undersized annular ring to improve leaflet apposition. Therefore, patients who are to undergo coronary artery bypass graft (CABG) surgery should be adequately assessed preoperatively for mitral regurgitation.

8

Mitral Valve Prolapse

CASE PRESENTATION

A 26-year old married woman visited a renowned cardiologist for coronary angiography, with the complaints of episodic chest pain and palpitation. The chest pain was precordial in location and described as sharp and pricking. There was no feeling of tightness in the chest or suffocation and the pain did not radiate to the left arm or lower jaw. The palpitation was accompanied by restlessness, dryness of mouth and dizziness and sometimes caused "black-out" with fainting. The episodes of chest pain and palpitation were unrelated to physical exercise, taking meals or change in body posture, but usually related to some emotional upheaval. She had first experienced these symptoms during her final high-school exams at the age of 18, but the frequency of episodes had significantly increased, ever since her arranged marriage 3 months back. There was history of repeated sore-throat during childhood, but she never had a prolonged febrile illness with painful joints.

On examination, the patient had a slender body habitus with an anxious look on her face. The extremities were warm with sweaty palms and a fine distal tremor. There was no anemia, cyanosis or edema and the JVP was not raised. The thyroid gland was not enlarged and there were no eye-signs of Grave's disease. The pulse was rapid, good in volume at a rate of 96 beats/min with a BP of 140/84 mm Hg. The precordium was hyperdynamic with a pectus excavatum sternal deformity. The apex beat was normal in location and there was no parasternal heave. The S_1 was loud, S_2 was normally split and no S_3 or S_4 was heard in diastole. A high-pitched systolic murmur was audible between the cardiac apex and the left sternal border. The murmur started well after the S_1 and had a typical honking character. It was associated with a sharp clicking sound in mid-systole. The lung fields were clear on auscultation.

CLINICAL DISCUSSION

From the history and physical examination, this young anxious lady had atypical cardiac symptoms with a mid-systolic click and a mid-systolic murmur. The most likely diagnosis in this case is mitral valve prolapse (MVP). The mid-systolic click is a high-pitched sharp sound produced by sudden tensing of the redundant mitral leaflet. At times, multiple clicks are appreciated. This is often followed by a mid- or late-systolic murmur that typically has a whooping or honking character.

Another cause of a mid-systolic murmur is papillary muscle dysfunction. The click and murmur can vary with alteration of left ventricular (LV) volume, by change in patient posture. During standing or Valsalva manoeuvre, when the LV volume is reduced, the click moves closer to S_1 and the murmur becomes louder. Conversely, during squatting when the LV volume increases, the click moves closer to S_2 and the murmur becomes softer.

In mitral valve prolapse syndrome, the S_1 is loud for several reasons. The high adrenergic activity increases the heart rate and shortens diastole. The wide excursion of the myxomatous, redundant valve leaflet increases the force of mitral valve closure. Finally, merger of the non-ejection click with the S_1, increases the intensity of the latter.

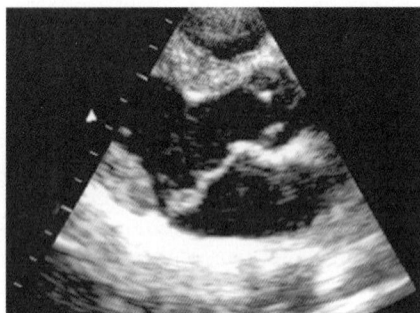

Figure 8.1: ECHO showing buckling of mitral leaflets, above the plane of mitral annulus

ECG of the patient showed sinus rhythm at the rate of 92 with few atrial ectopic beats and T wave inversion in leads L_{III}, aVF, V_5, V_6. The X-ray chest was unremarkable. On ECHO, the left ventricle was normal in size and systolic function, but the left atrium was mildly dilated. The anterior mitral leaflet was thick and redundant, with systolic buckling above the plane of the mitral annulus into the left atrium (Fig. 8.1). On M-Mode scan, there was abrupt posterior displacement of both leaflets in systole, giving a "hammock-like" appearance (Fig. 8.2). On colour flow mapping, an eccentric regurgitant jet was seen entering the left atrium.

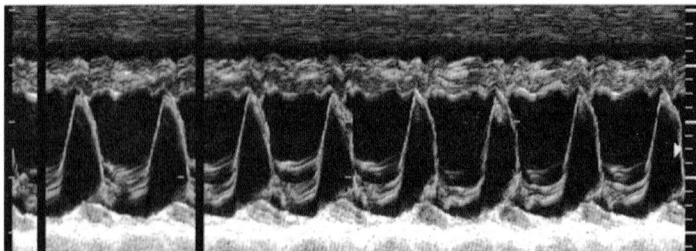

Figure 8.2: M-mode scan showing posterior motion of mitral leaflets ("hammock" appearance)

According to the extent of motion, mitral valve prolapse (MVP) can be classified into 3 types (Table 8.1). In type 1, the anterior leaflet only moves upto the annulus while in type 2, it bows into the left atrium. In type 3, both the leaflets enter the left atrium. Strict echocardiographic criteria must be used to diagnose MVP because needless anxiety may be created by over-reporting this abnormality. Minor "technical" MVP may be observed in normal women due to high transducer position and caudal angulation. Conversely, true MVP may be missed due to low transducer position and cranial angulation.

Table 8.1: Classification of mitral valve prolapse
Type 1: AML and PML move upto the annulus
Type 2: Large AML bows into the left atrium
Type 3: Both AML and PML enter left atrium

Mitral valve prolapse is known as "floppy valve" or "myxomatous valve" or "billowing valve" and the condition is also designated as "Barlow's syndrome". MVP is far more commonly seen in females and occurs in 7% of middle-aged women. Often these women have a type A personality with history of panic attacks and migranous headaches. They may have a slender body habitus with thoracic skeletal deformities including pectus excavatum, straight back and scoliosis. The valvular abnormality is due to myxomatous degeneration leading to thickening, nodularity or redundancy of one or both mitral leaflets. Sometimes MVP is associated with other cardiac conditions such as ostium seundum ASD, Marfan syndrome and WPW syndrome (Table 8.2). Mitral regurgitation may be present due to faulty coaptation of leaflets and predisposes to endocarditis.

Table 8.2: Conditions associated with MVP
• Myxomatous degeneration
• Rheumatic heart disease
• Ostium secundum ASD
• WPW syndrome
• Marfan syndrome
• Turner syndrome

Atypical chest pain, palpitation, fatigue, orthostatic symptoms and neuro-psychiatric complaints have all been well-described in patients with mitral valve prolapse. Whether these non-specific symptoms are directly attributable to MVP or due to autonomic dysfunction, continues to be widely debated and their cause-effect relationship remains unproven. Besides the classical symptoms, focal neurologic findings, such as transient ischemic attacks, amaurosis fugax, retinal artery occlusion and rarely hemiparesis have all been reported in patients with MVP. These neurologic findings probably occur as a result of thrombo-embolism from the prolapsing valve.

The ECG at rest frequently shows T-wave inversion in the inferolateral leads (L_{III}, aVF, V_5, V_6). False-positive ECG stress tests occur in up to 50% of patients with MVP. Premature beats are most common, although practically any arrhythmia can occur. The cause of the arrhythmia is not known but may be related to autonomic dysfunction or mechanical effects of the floppy valve. Incidence of syncope correlates poorly with the presence of arrhythmias.

PERTINENT INVESTIGATIONS

It is not unusual for patients of mitral valve prolapse to undergo a battery of sophisticated cardiac investigations, in the search for the diagnosis of a serious heart disease. Besides ECG and ECHO which do show some typical abnormalities, exercise stress test is done which is more often false-positive. Ambulatory 24-hour Holter monitoring frequently shows supraventricular and sometimes ventricular ectopic beats and rarely if ever reveals life-threatening arrhythmias. Myocardial perfusion imaging and coronary angiography expectedly do not show any significant abnormality. Hormonal assays are sometimes performed to rule out thyrotoxicosis and likewise, urinary catecholamines are rarely measured, to rule out the possibility of phaeochromocytoma.

MANAGEMENT ISSUES

Most women with mitral valve prolapse need reassurance that their cardiac condition is not serious or life-threatening. Anxiolytic drugs during the day with a mild tranquilizer at night are useful for those having overt anxiety and disturbed sleep. A beta-blocker such as propranolol has multiple benefits in these patients. It controls tachycardia and ectopic beats, reduces the degree of leaflet prolapse, treats the associated tremor and serves as a prophylactic drug against migraine. Low-dose aspirin is prescribed to prevent thrombo-embolism. Patients of MVP with mitral regurgitation (MR) and not those without demonstrable MR, require antibiotic prophylaxis against infective endocarditis, prior to a dental, endoscopic or surgical procedure.

Aortic Valve Diseases

Aortic Stenosis

CASE PRESENTATION

A 52-year old man presented to the out-patient cardiology clinic with easy fatiguability and breathlessness on exertion for the last 1 year. In the preceding month, he had experienced three distinct episodes of dizziness, followed by fainting. The syncopal episodes were unrelated to exercise and were not preceded by palpitation or chest pain. There was no history of prolonged febrile illness or joint pains during childhood.

On examination, the pulse was of low volume with a slow upstroke, at a rate of 84 beats/min. with a BP of 96/72 mm Hg. There was no anemia, cyanosis or icterus and the thyroid gland was not enlarged. The JVP was not raised and there was no ankle edema. The apex beat was normal in position and heaving in nature. The S_1 was normal, S_2 appeared single and S_4 was audible in pre-systole. An ejection systolic murmur was audible over the aortic area, that was preceded by an ejection click and associated with a palpable thrill. The murmur and thrill typically radiated towards the carotid arteries.

CLINICAL DISCUSSION

From the history and physical examination, this man had low cardiac output, possibly due to left ventricular outflow tract (LVOT) obstruction. The most likely diagnosis in this case is aortic valve stenosis (Fig. 9.1). A pulse of low volume (pulsus parvus) with slow upstroke (pulsus tardus) is a typical feature of aortic valve stenosis. A heaving apex beat indicates left ventricular hypertrophy and is also observed in uncontrolled systemic hypertension and in coarctation of aorta.

The low-pitched S_4 sound in pre-systole, indicates forceful atrial contraction over a non-compliant left ventricle. It coincides with the *a* wave of the jugular vein. The S_4 is always pathological in aortic stenosis, systemic hypertension and restrictive or hypertrophic cardiomyopathy. An acute rise in left ventricular end-diastolic pressure (LVEDP) as in acute coronary syndrome or acute valvular regurgitation causes acute onset of S_4.

The S_2 appears single because the A_2 is muffled. If A_2 is audible, the splitting of S_2 is paradoxical or reverse, with the A_2 following the P_2 due to prolonged left ventricular ejection time. The ejection click heralds the onset of systole and the end of isovolumic relaxation. It indicates that the stenosis is valvular in nature

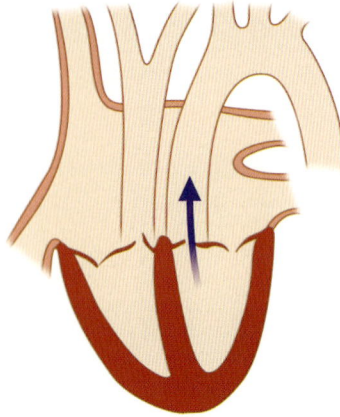

Figure 9.1: Aortic valve stenosis

and not subvalvular (infundibular) in location. The click may be absent if the valve is heavily calcified. The ejection systolic murmur of aortic stenosis indicates turbulent flow across the narrow aortic valve orifice. It is described as a diamond-shaped murmur, since it builds up and declines gradually, with maximal intensity in mid-systole. This pattern coincides with the temporal profile of the pressure gradient across the valve. This murmur is also described as a "crescendo-decrescendo murmur". Length and loudness of the murmur does not correlate with the severity of aortic stenosis.

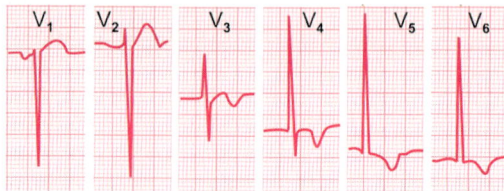

Figure 9.2: ECG showing tall R waves in lateral chest leads

ECG showed tall R waves in left precordial leads with T wave inversion, indicative of left ventricular hypertrophy with strain (Fig. 9.2). X-ray chest findings were a boot-shaped heart with a prominent ascending aorta, suggestive of post-stenotic dilatation. On ECHO, the left ventricular cavity was small in size, with a good ejection fraction. There was concentric thickening of the interventricular septum (IVS) and the left ventricular posterior wall (LVPW). The aortic valve leaflets were thickened and calcific with restricted excursion and reduced opening of the valve. Due to fusion at the leaflet tips, there was systolic doming of leaflets. On colour flow mapping, a mosaic jet was observed in the proximal aorta (Fig. 9.3) with an increased systolic velocity across the valve on CW Doppler.

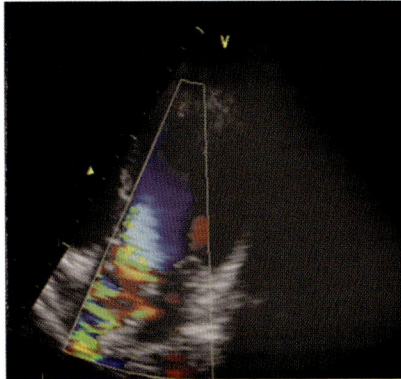

Figure 9.3: ECHO showing a mosaic colored jet
in the proximal aorta

Table 9.1: Assessment of the severity of aortic stenosis			
	Mild	**Moderate**	**Severe**
V_{max} (m/sec)	<2.5	2.5-4	>4
PG (mm Hg)	<2.5	25-60	>60
AVa (cm²)	>1.5	1.0-1.5	<1.0
Vmax : Peak velocity PG : Pressure gradient AVa : Aortic valve area			

Transthoracic echocardiography (TEE) generally suffices for the diagnosis of aortic stenosis. However, the severity of stenosis is determined from the peak velocity and pressure gradient across the valve on Doppler (Table 9.1). Measurements from various echo views are taken to obtain the peak aortic flow velocity. In rheumatic aortic stenosis, assessment of concomitant mitral valve abnormalities is crucial as the mitral valve is almost invariably involved. Finally, left ventricular wall thickness, end-diastolic diameter and ejection fraction are to be measured. There are some fallacies associated with the calculation of aortic stenosis severity. Reverberation artifacts in a heavily calcified valve may overestimate AS severity. The peak velocity and pressure gradient depend on the heart rate and stroke volume. They also depend upon the degree of parallelism obtained between the Doppler beam and aortic flow direction.

Table 9.2: Causes of aortic stenosis
• Congenital bicuspid valve
• Rheumatic heart disease
• Senile calcific degeneration

The main causes of AS are congenital bicuspid aortic valve, rheumatic heart disease and senile calcific degeneration (Table 9.2). Rheumatic aortic stenosis usually presents in the 2nd or 3rd decade of life and is almost always associated with mitral valve disease. Congenital bicuspid aortic valve leads to aortic stenosis because of increased mechanical and shear stress on the valve and usually presents in the 4th of 5th decade. Calcific aortic stenosis is akin to atherosclerosis and accompanied by multiple cardiovascular risk factors. It typically presents in the 6th or 7th decade of life. Rarely, a discrete membrane or ring may cause subvalvular or supravalvular AS. Complications of AS are left ventricular hypertrophy with diastolic dysfunction earlier on and systolic heart failure in the later stages. Syncopal episodes are due to tachyarrhythmias or LVOT obstruction. Angina may occur because of coronary ostial stenosis or the increased oxygen demand of the hypertrophied myocardium.

PERTINENT INVESTIGATIONS

Exercise ECG testing and Dobutamine stress ECHO may be undertaken in asymptomatic patients of aortic stenosis, to assess their functional capacity. The characteristic response is a drop in blood pressure during the test due to vasodilatation and failure of the cardiac output to rise. Patients with a positive test may be taken up for valve replacement. Coronary angiography is indicated to assess the coronary circulation and need by bypass graft surgery (CABG), at the time of aortic valve replacement. Besides showing occlusive coronary disease, angiography may reveal coronary ostial stenosis due to calcification of the aortic valve.

MANAGEMENT ISSUES

There is no medical treatment for aortic stenosis barring perhaps low-does aspirin with a statin in those who have associated coronary risk factors. Aortic valve replacement (AVR) is the procedure of choice in symptomatic severe aortic stenosis or in asymptomatic stenosis with left ventricular dysfunction or a positive stress test. AVR may also be undertaken in moderate AS at the time of CABG surgery or in those engaged in high profile jobs such as aircraft pilots or military personnel (Table 9.3). Complications of aortic valve replacement are prosthetic valve malfunction, thrombo-embolism or bleeding and infective endocarditis.

Table 9.3: Indications for surgery in aortic stenosis
• Moderate to severe AS with symptoms
• Moderate AS with a positive stress test
• Moderate to severe AS with LV dysfunction
• Moderate AS with high profile job (e.g. pilot)
• Moderate AS with planned surgery (e.g. CABG)

RECENT ADVANCES

The technique of percutaneous aortic valve replacement (AVR) has been recently refined and its feasibility is now clearly established. It is particular suitable for candidates at high risk for a surgical procedure under general anesthesia. The role of percutaneous aortic balloon valvuloplasty is currently limited.

C A S E

10

Aortic
Regurgitation

CASE PRESENTATION

A 54-year old man presented with breathlessness on exertion and throbbing headache. His exertional dyspnea started about 8 months back and progressed to the extent that he found it difficult to climb even one flight of stairs. His throbbing headache was a daily feature and he also felt some pulsations over the neck. There was no history of exertional chest pain, palpitation or syncopal episodes. The patient had visited an orthopedician for a still back with difficulty in bending forward. On X-ray of the lumbo-sacral spine, it was diagnosed as ankylosing spondylitis. He was taking oral steroids prescribed by an ophthalmologist for iridocyclitis, in addition to his antihypertensive medication.

On examination, the radial pulse was of good volume and bounding in nature at a rate of 84 beats/min. The BP was 160/64 mm Hg in the right arm. Pulsations were visible over the carotid arteries and the femoral pulses were also bounding in nature. There was no clinical sign of congestive heart failure. The apex beat was diffuse and hyperkinetic in nature and significantly displaced towards the axilla. The S_1 was normal and the S_2 was soft, with a S_3 gallop sound in early diastole. A high-pitched blowing murmur was heard in diastole soon after the S_3, on either side of the upper sternum. A short diastolic rumble was also heard over the cardiac apex. Few scattered crepts were audible over the lower lung fields.

CLINICAL DISCUSSION

From the history and physical examination, this man had aortic regurgitation (Fig. 10.1) with possibly mitral stenosis and evidence of left ventricular dilatation. Aortic root dilatation with AR is a known complication of ankylosing spondylitis. The early-diastolic decrescendo murmur of AR is soft and blowing in character, best heard with the patient sitting up and leaning forward. Interestingly, when AR is due to aortic root dilatation, the murmur is louder along the right sternal border. When AR is due to aortic valve pathology, the murmur is louder along the left sternal border. In acute AR, for instance due to dissection of aorta, the murmur is very short and soft and associated with a S_4 and not S_3.

The diastolic rumble at the apex does not necessary indicate concomitant mitral stenosis. It is due to fluttering of the anterior mitral leaflet between the AR jet and mitral valve inflow and is known as Austin-Flint murmur. A bounding

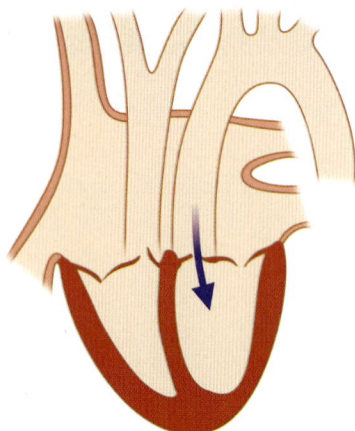

Figure 10.1: Aortic regurgitation

("water-hammer") pulse that can be appreciated even with the arm elevated above the head is known as a collapsing pulse and is indicative of a wide pulse-pressure. Besides aortic regurgitation, causes of wide pulse pressure are severe anemia, thyrotoxicosis, beri-beri disease, patent ductus arteriosus and arteriovenous fistula. Certain classical clinical signs of wide pulse-pressure, have been described in aortic regurgitation (Table 10.1).

Table 10.1: Clinical signs of aortic regurgitation	
• Corrigan sign:	Vigorous pulsations in the carotid vessels
• De Musset sign:	Nodding of the head with each heart beat
• Quincke sign:	Visible capillary pulsations in the nail bed
• Traube sign:	Pistol-shot sounds over femoral arteries
• Duroziez sign:	Diastolic murmur over femoral arteries

ECG of the patient showed tall R waves in left precordial leads with upright T waves indicating left ventricular diastolic overload. X-ray chest findings were cardiomegaly and pulmonary congestion, giving it a "bat-wing" appearance (Fig. 10.2). On ECHO, the left ventricle was dilated with an ejection fraction of 45%. There was also dilatation of the aortic root but the aortic valve leaflets were not thickened or calcific and had no vegetations. The mitral valve was structurally normal and the left atrium was normal in size. On colour flow mapping, a regurgitant jet was seen entering the left ventricular outflow tract (Fig. 10.3). The volume of AR (ml/beat), the width of the AR jet as percentage of LVOT diameter (%) and the depth of the jet entry into the left ventricle are used to gauge the severity of AR (Table 10.2). However, there are some fallacies associated with these calculations. The narrow jet of mild AR may extend deep into the left ventricle while the broad jet of severe AR may not extend that far if it is "eccentric" or "off-centre".

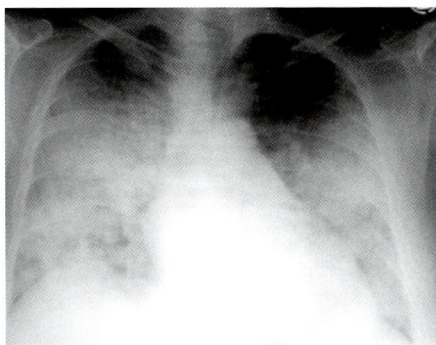

Figure 10.2: X-ray showing cardiomegaly
with pulmonary congestion

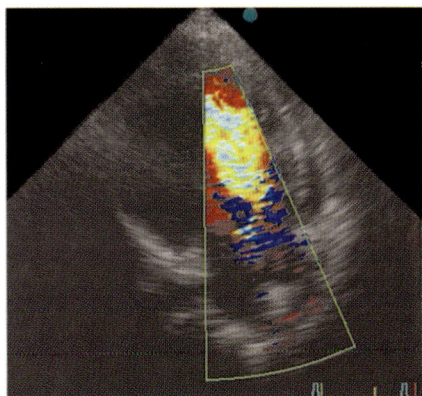

Figure 10.3: ECHO showing regurgitant jet
in the outflow tract

Table 10.2: Assessment of the severity of aortic regurgitation			
	Mild	**Moderate**	**Severe**
AR jet depth upto	LVOT	Mid–LV	LV apex
AR jet width (% of LVOT)	<25	25-65	>65
AR volume (ml/beat)	<30	30-59	>60
AR: Aortic regurgitation on Doppler LVOT: Left ventricular outflow tract			

The causes of aortic regurgitation can be classified into the causes of aortic valve disease and the causes of aortic root dilatation. Valvular diseases are congenital bicuspid aortic valve, rheumatic heart disease and connective tissue disorders. Aortic root dilatation occurs in uncontrolled hypertension, Marfan's syndrome and ankylosing spondylitis. Acute AR can result from aortic dissection, annulo–aortic ectasia, infective endocarditis or after blunt trauma to the chest (Table 10.3).

Table 10.3: Causes of aortic regurgitation
Valvular AR
• Bicuspid aortic valve
• Rheumatic heart disease
• Connective tissue disorder
Root dilatation
• Marfan syndrome
• Ankylosing spondylitis
• Systemic hypertension
Acute AR
• Chest wall trauma
• Dissection of aorta
• Infective endocarditis

PERTINENT INVESTIGATIONS

In addition to echocardiography, cardiac computed tomography (CT) or magnetic resonance imaging (MRI) may be required for the detailed assessment of the aortic valve as well as the proximal aorta. Radionuclide ventriculography may be required for the detailed assessment of left ventricular volume, geometry and systolic function. Exercise testing may be considered in an asymptomatic person to assess his functional capacity. Coronary angiography is indicated to assess the coronary circulation and the need for bypass surgery at the time of aortic valve replacement. At the time of angiography, a root aortogram should also be performed to assess the proximal aorta.

MANAGEMENT ISSUES

As far as the medical management of AR is concerned, diuretics and vasodilators are the mainstay of therapy. The diuretics reduce blood pressure, left ventricular volume and the symptoms of heart failure. Vasodilators reduce afterload, increase forward flow and decrease the regurgitant volume. Additionally, they control systolic blood pressure which is nearly always an issue in these patients. Aortic valve replacement (AVR) is the surgical procedure of choice in patients of AR who are symptomatic or have left ventricular dilatation (Table 10.4). Aortic root repair or replacement may be combined with AVR, if there is a significant degree of aortic dilatation. AVR may be combined with coronary artery bypass graft (CABG) surgery, if the latter is indicated.

Table 10.4: Indications for surgery in aortic regurgitation		
• Symptomatic acute moderate to severe AR		
• Symptomatic chronic moderate to severe AR		
• Asymptomatic chronic AR of any degree with left ventricular dysfunction and dilatation		
LV dilatation	:	end-systolic diameter >55 mm end-diastolic diameter >75 mm
LV dysfunction	:	LV ejection fraction <50%

RECENT ADVANCES

Aortic valve replacement with a mechanical or a bioprosthetic valve is associated with either the need for a long-term anticoagulant (requires monitoring and carries risk of bleeding) or the late failure of a bioprosthetic valve. Therefore, there is now growing interest in aortic valve repair, if the valvular anatomy is suitable. However, the long-term feasability of this technique needs further evaluation.

11

Aortic Sclerosis

CASE PRESENTATION

A 77-year old elderly gentleman was brought by his son to his regular physician, for a routine periodic medical check-up. The patient had been hypertensive for the last 35 years and presently he was taking amlodipine 5 mg and metoprolol 50 mg daily. About 3 years back, he was also prescribed isosorbide mononitrate 40 mg and aspirin 75mg daily, because his ECG showed T wave inversion in the lateral leads. The patient did complain of breathlessness on climbing stairs but there was no history of angina, orthopnea or paroxysmal nocturnal dyspnea. Over the last three months, he also felt dizzy and light-headed on standing up from the lying position, but there was no history of palpitation or syncope.

On examination, the pulse was of good volume with few missed beats and the BP was 154/76 mm Hg, with a heart rate of 66 beats/min. The patient was conscious, cooperative and in no distress. The JVP was not raised but there was minimal pitting edema over both his ankles. The apex beat was slightly displaced towards the axilla and heaving in character. Systolic pulsations were observed over the aortic area and in the suprasternal notch. The S_1 was normal, A_2 was loud but no gallop was audible. A harsh systolic murmur was heard over the upper left sternal edge that radiated towards the neck. The murmur was not preceded by an ejection click or accompanied by a palpable thrill. A different soft systolic murmur was heard over the cardiac apex that radiated towards the left axilla. The lung fields were clear on auscultation.

CLINICAL DISCUSSION

From the history and physical examination, this elderly hypertensive gentleman had aortic root dilatation, with probably left ventricular outflow tract (LVOT) obstruction and also mitral regurgitation. ECG showed tall R waves with inverted T waves in the lateral precordial leads (Fig. 11.1). There were no significant Q waves or S-T segment shift, but few unifocal ventricular premature beats were observed. X-ray chest findings were mild cardiomegaly, dilated ascending aorta and a prominent aortic knuckle (Fig. 11.2).

ECHO revealed normal sized left ventricular cavity, with an ejection fraction of 45%. There was mild concentric hypertrophy, but no wall motion abnormality of any ventricular segment. The aortic valve annulus and leaflets showed bright

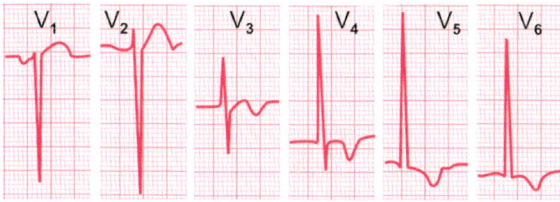

Figure 11.1: ECG showing tall R waves with inverted T waves in lateral leads

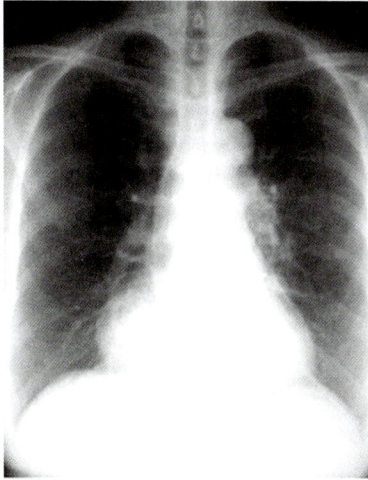

Figure 11.2: X-ray showing dilated ascending aorta with prominent aortic knuckle

echo-reflectivity (Fig. 11.3) with some restriction of leaflet excursion, but no systolic doming. The posterior segment of the mitral valve annulus and the base of the posterior leaflet also showed high echogenicity. On colour flow mapping, a mosaic jet was seen entering the left atrium across the mitral valve. On Doppler study, a peak systolic velocity (Vmax) of 2.5 m/sec was seen across the aortic valve with a calculated pressure gradient (PG) of 25 mm Hg.

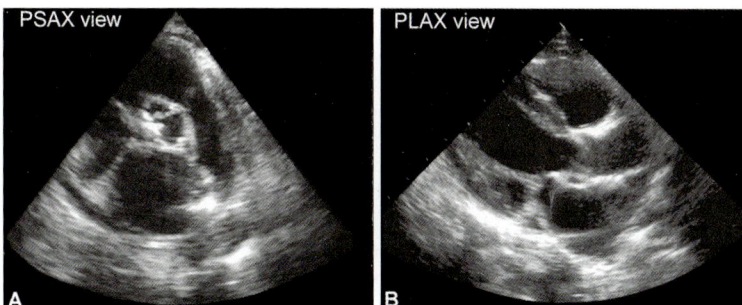

Figure 11.3: ECHO showing calcification of aortic valve leaflets (A) and annulus (B)

Table 11.1: Causes of aortic root dilatation	
• Post-stenotic	Aortic stenosis
• Medial necrosis	Marfan's syndrome
• Aorto-arteritis	Takayasu's disease
• Atherosclerotic	Elderly hypertensive
• Collagen disorder	Ankylosing spondylitis

Dilatation of the proximal aorta or aortic root is not uncommon in elderly hypertensive subjects due to atherosclerosis. The aortic valve annulus however, is normal in diameter. Aortic dilatation also occurs in aortic valve stenosis due to the high velocity jet through the narrow, distorted valve impinging on the aortic wall. This is known as post-stenotic dilatation. Sometimes, aortic root dilatation is due to medial necrosis (Marfan's syndrome), aorto-arteritis (Takayasu's disease) or a connective tissue disorder (Ankylosing spondylitis). In these cases, the aortic valve annulus is also dilated and aortic regurgitation is often associated (Table 11.1).

In elderly hypertensive patients, besides aortic root dilatation, calcification of the aortic valve with or without stenosis is sometimes observed. This entity is referred to as aortic valve sclerosis. Aortic valve calcification may also be accompanied by mitral annular calcification (MAC). The calcified mitral annulus sometimes causes mild to moderate mitral regurgitation and rarely even mitral stenosis. Aortic sclerosis occurs in 25% subjects above the age of 65 years. It leads to aortic stenosis more often in those about 80 years of age with a severely calcified valve and in the presence of chronic kidney disease. There is a 50% risk of myocardial infarction, stroke or death within 5 years, due to multiple cardiovascular risk factors and severe atherosclerosis.

The systolic murmur of aortic stenosis is sometimes preceded by an ejection click, accompanied by a palpable thrill and followed by a muffled A_2 due to reduced ejection volume. On the other hand, with the murmur of aortic sclerosis, there is no click or thrill and the A_2 is loud because of associated systemic hypertension. A history of dizziness or syncope should always altert us to the possibility of left ventricular outflow tract (LVOT) obstruction. Alternatively, syncope can occur due to a tachyarrhythmia or because of sinus node dysfunction. In a patient of aortic sclerosis, angina pectoris may be multifactorial. One, there may be coronary artery stenosis. Two, the calcification of the valve may cause coronary ostial occlusion. Three, angina may be due to the increased myocardial oxygen demand, as a consequence of left ventricular hypertrophy.

MANAGEMENT ISSUES

The medical management of aortic valve sclerosis includes adequate control of hypertension and other cardiovascular risk factors. This patient was already taking amlodipine and metoprolol. Ramipril may be added since it is known to facilitate regression of left ventricular hypertrophy. Diuretics should be avoided if there is history of syncope. A statin can be added to the ongoing aspirin since both these agents are proven to prevent cardiovascular events. Elderly hypertensive patients often have associated orthostatic symptoms and they should be advised adequate fluid intake and gradual change of posture.

Aortic valve replacement (AVR) may be considered in symptomatic moderate to severe aortic stenosis especially with left ventricular dysfunction. At the time of AVR, coronary angiography should be performed to assess the status of the coronary vasculature. Conversely, all patients to be taken up for coronary artery bypass graft (CABG) surgery should be assessed for aortic stenosis and AVR can be performed at the time of operation.

RECENT ADVANCES

The technique of percutaneous aortic valve replacement (AVR) has been recently refined and it is now clearly feasible in candidates at high risk of a surgical procedure under general anesthesia.

The Cardiomyopathies

12

Dilated Cardiomyopathy

CASE PRESENTATION

A 48-year old man presented to the emergency room with recent worsening of breathlessness, over the past few days. His dyspnea was worse at night and he required two or more pillows under his head to catch some sleep. Yet his nocturnal breathlessness woke him up frequently. For the past 4 months he had experienced increasing fatigue on walking and on climbing stairs. He was not a diabetic or hypertensive and denied any chest pain, palpitation or syncope. He did not smoke but took 5-6 large pegs of alcohol on most days of the week, for the last 30 years. None of his family members had history of heart disease.

On examination, he was tachypneic and diaphoretic. Pulse was rapid and feeble with a changing volume in alternate beats and the extremities were cold. His heart rate was 120 beats/min with a BP of 106/74 mm Hg. The JVP was clearly elevated and there was also pitting edema over his ankles. The liver edge was palpable 6 cm below the right costal margin. The apex beat was diffuse and displaced towards the axilla. The S_1 and S_2 were normal and there was a soft pansystolic murmur over the mitral area with an audible gallop sound in early diastole. There were bilateral basilar rales over the lower one-third of both lung fields.

CLINICAL DISCUSSION

Form the history and physical examination, this patient was obviously in congestive cardiac failure. The heart failure was systolic in nature, of the low-output variety and biventricular in origin. ECG showed sinus tachycardia, narrow QRS complexes and non-specific T-wave inversion, without any S-T segment shift or Q-waves. X-ray chest findings were moderate cardiomegaly, Kerley B lines, hilar congestion, and cephalized vessels, with pulmonary edema and a small right-sided pleural effusion (Fig. 12.1). ECHO revealed a dilated left ventricle (ejection fraction 25-30%) with reduced septal and posterior wall motion (global hypokinesia). Excursion of the mitral valve leaflets was decreased and the E-point septal separation was increased (Fig. 12.2). There were no regional wall motion abnormalities or abnormal architecture of the cardiac valves. There was mild mitral regurgitation and mild right ventricular dilatation. There are three main diagnostic possibilities in this case. These are:

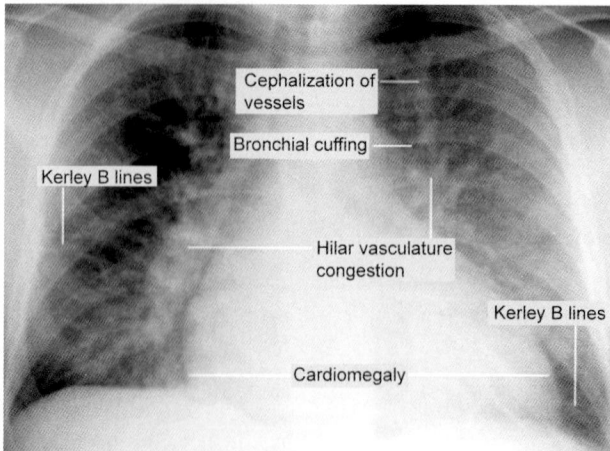

Figure 12.1: X-ray showing the classical findings of left ventricular systolic dysfunction

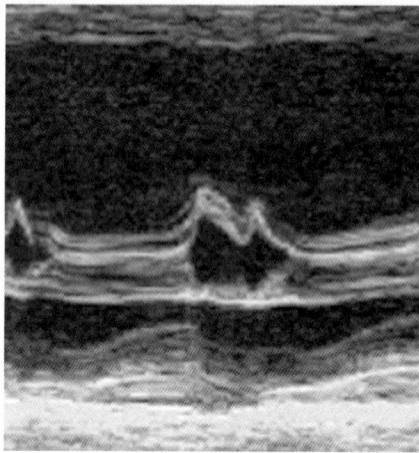

Figure 12.2: ECHO showing reduced excursion of the septum and mitral leaflets

- Organic mitral regurgitation
- Ischemic cardiomyopathy
- Dilated cardiomyopathy.

Organic mitral regurgitation with volume overload leading to severe left ventricular dysfunction is unlikely in this case, because the mitral valve architecture was normal and valvular regurgitation was only mild in severity. Ischemic cardiomyopathy is a diagnostic possibility, but there are several reasons against it. The patient had no significant coronary risk factors or family history of heart disease. ECG did not show any S-T segment shift or the presence of Q-waves. On ECHO, there was global hypokinesia instead of regional wall motion abnormality. Moreover, there were no dyskinetic segments in the left ventricular

Table 12.1: Differences between dilated and ischemic cardiomyopathy		
	Dilated CMP	**Ischemic CMP**
Hypokinesia	Global	Regional
RWMA and the coronary territory	Do not conform	Conform
Dyskinesia	Not seen	Seen
RV involvement	Often	Rare

wall while right ventricular dilatation was present (Table 12.1). Therefore, the most probable diagnosis in this case is dilated cardiomyopathy.

There are several causes of dilated cardiomyopathy (DCMP). The idiopathic variety is believed to follow an acute viral myocarditis. Prominent definite causes of DCMP are heavy alcoholism, diabetes mellitus and the peri-partum period. Familial DCMP is seen in Duchenne's muscular dystrophy and Friedrich's ataxia. Deficiency of thiamine (vitamin B_1), selenium and carnitine can cause a reversible form of DCMP. Drugs implicated in the causation of DCMP are doxorubicin, imatinib, cyclophosphamide and trastuzumab. Uncommonly, a persistent tachycardia due to any cause, can lead to permanent DCMP (Table 12.2).

Table 12.2: Causes of dilated cardiomyopathy
• Idiopathic
• Alcoholism
• Diabetes
• Peripartum
• Nutritional
• Drug induced
• Tachycardia related

PERTINENT INVESTIGATIONS

While echocardiography is a dependable diagnostic modality for dilated cardiomyopathy, a battery of tests can be performed to ascertain the etiological diagnosis. This is because there are several causes of DCMP and a vigorous search is warranted to identify a treatable cause, with the optimism of preventing relentless progression of the disease.

Inflammatory markers (ESR and CRP) are elevated in the presence of myocarditis while levels of biomarkers (CPK, LDH) are increased in myocardial necrosis. Patients are screened for a chronic infection (HIV, Hepatitis C) or nutritional deficiency (thiamine, selenium, carnitine). Serum iron, ferritin and transferrin are ordered if anemia or hemochromatosis are suspected and T_3, T_4 and TSH if thyrotoxicosis is to be ruled out. Renal and liver function tests are ordered to assess additional causes of fluid overload.

Cardiac magnetic resonance imaging (MRI) is useful to assess left ventricular size and geometry, LV remodelling and for tissue characterization with gadolinium enhancement. Coronary angiography is performed in the presence of atherosclerotic risk factors. Endomyocardial biopsy is rarely performed because of its low diagnostic yield.

MANAGEMENT ISSUES

The first step in the management of DCMP is to identify and treat reversible factors. Measures include withdrawal of the offending drug and correction of any nutritional deficiency. Abstinence from alcohol and control of diabetes are equally important. The heart rate has to be controlled in tachycardia related cardiomyopathy.

Treatment of most of these patients is on the lines of standard heart failure therapy. Diuretics are prescribed to treat fluid overload and modulators of renin-angiotensin system (ACE-inhibitors or ARBs) to reduce cardiac afterload. Beta-blockers are used particularly if extreme tachycardia or atrial fibrillation are present. If the patient has persistent atrial fibrillation, rate control with digoxin is required. Additionally, the patients are initiated on an oral anticoagulant to reduce the risk of thrombo-embolic complications.

RECENT ADVANCES

A significant proportion of patients with dilated cardiomyopathy succumb to malignant ventricular arrhythmias and not to heart failure per se. Antiarrhythmic drugs reduce ejection fraction and have proarrhythmic potential, besides their systemic side-effects. The use of automatic implantable cardioverter defibrilla-tors (AICDs) is now advocated as a primary preventive strategy against sudden cardiac death (SCD) in such patients. Anticoagulant therapy is widely prescribed to patients who are in atrial fibrillation and in those where a mural thrombus has been documented. Currently, trials are underway to evaluate the role of anticoagulants against thromboembolic complications in patients who are in sinus rhythm.

In patients with moderate to severe symptoms (NYHA Class III or IV) with severe left ventricular dysfunction (LVEF below 30%) and wide QRS complexes (QRS duration more than 120 msec), cardiac resynchronization therapy (CRT) may be offered. A biventricular pacemaker is placed to synchronize the ejection of right and left ventricles if there is left bundle branch block (LBBB) or an intraventricular conduction defect (IVCD). Finally, a ventricular assist device may be implanted to improve left ventricular function in those with significant hemodynamic deterioration. This strategy is particularly useful as a bridge to cardiac transplantation.

13

Restrictive Cardiomyopathy

CASE PRESENTATION

A 58-year old man presented to the cardiology facility with fatigue, difficulty in breathing and increasing swelling over his ankles, for the last 3 months. His dyspnea became worse at night and he required two or more pillows under his head to be comfortable. In addition, he had noticed an increase in his abdominal girth and had loss of appetite, but there was no weight loss. There was no history of fever, productive cough, chest pain or hemoptysis. He also denied palpitations or episodes of syncope. The patient was not hypertensive or diabetic and there was no history of premature coronary artery disease in any of his family members.

On examination, he was tachypneic but not in any distress. The pulse was 90 beats /min with a BP of 114/72 mm Hg. There was no cyanosis or jaundice but pitting edema was present around the ankles. The liver edge was palpable 6 cm below the right costal margin and there was free fluid in the abdominal cavity. The JVP was elevated 5 cm above the angle of Louis, with prominent *a* waves and without a fall in its level during inspiration. The apex beat was normal in character and location, without any displacement towards the axilla. The S_1 and S_2 were normal with an audible S_4 in late diastole. There was no murmur or pericardial friction rub. Crepts were audible over the basilar lung fields posteriorly.

CLINICAL DISCUSSION

From the history and physical examination, this patient was clearly having biventricular heart failure. ECG showed low QRS voltages with non-specific T-wave changes but no Q waves. There was no tachyarrhythmia or conduction block. X-ray chest findings were interstitial pulmonary edema and small bilateral pleural effusion, but the heart size was normal. ECHO revealed relative small ventricular chambers with bilateral atrial dilatation. The ventricular free walls and the interventricular septum were thick and gave a "granular sparkling" ground-glass appearance (Fig. 13.1). There was also thickening of the mitral and tricuspid valve leaflets with minimal valvular regurgitation. The left ventricular ejection fraction was normal but the transmitral Doppler showed a tall E-wave with rapid deceleration and a small A-wave.

There were several unusual clinical findings in this case. There was biventricular heart failure but no clinical or radiological evidence of cardiomegaly.

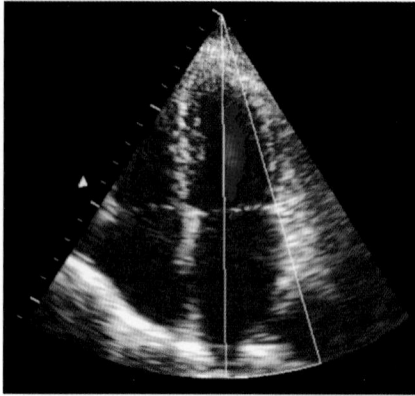

Figure 13.1: ECHO showing bright echogenicity
with small ventricles and large atria

Prominent *a* waves in the JVP and presence of S_4 on auscultation indicate atrial contraction against a stiff, noncompliant right ventricle. Failure of the JVP to fall during inspiration (or paradoxical rise) constitutes the Kussmaul's sign and also indicates ventricular diastolic restriction. Despite evidence of ventricular hypertrophy on ECHO, the voltages of the QRS complexes on the ECG were low. This indicates that myocardial infiltration was the cause of ventricular thickening in this case and not myocardial hypertrophy, as is observed in systemic hypertension and aortic stenosis. ECHO revealed relatively small ventricles and large atria, findings that are typically seen in mitral stenosis with pulmonary hypertension and secondary tricuspid regurgitation. However, in our case there was no evidence of mitral stenosis.

This patient therefore has a restrictive ventricular filling abnormality or left ventricular diastolic dysfunction (LVDD) or heart failure with preserved ejection fraction (HFPEF). Clinically speaking, the most frequent causes of LVDD are systemic hypertension and coronary artery disease, where the mitral inflow Doppler signal shows a slow relaxation pattern with the E wave shorter than the A wave. These conditions were clearly absent in our case. Therefore, the most probable diagnosis in this case is restrictive cardiomyopathy.

There are several causes of restrictive cardiomyopathy (RCMP). The most prominent cause of RCMP is endomyocardial fibrosis (EMF). Another reason is hypereosinophilic syndrome, the so called Loeffler's endocarditis. A variety of systemic infiltrative disease such as amyloidosis, sarcoidosis and malignancy can present with RCMP. Connective tissue disorders especially scleroderma can also lead to myocardial restriction. Finally, RCMP may be observed in storage diseases like hemochromatosis and glycogen storage disorders (Table 13.1).

Amyloidosis is an important cause of restrictive cardiomyopathy. Besides cardiac involvement, there may be other systemic manifestations of amyloid deposition. Macroglossia with periorbital ecchymosis is pathognomic of amyloidosis. Neurological manifestations are sensory neuropathy, carpal tunnel syndrome and autonomic neuropathy with postural hypotension. Hepatomegaly may be due to amyloid infiltration or due to congestive heart failure. Renal

Table 13.1: Causes of restrictive cardiomyopathy
Endomyocardial
Endomyocardial fibrosis
Hypereosinophilic syndrome
Infiltrative
Amyloidosis
Sarcoidosis
Malignancy
Gaucher's disease
Non-infiltrative
Idiopathic
Scleroderma
Storage diseases
Hemochromatosis
Glycogen storage disorder

involvement may lead to nephrotic syndrome, which exacerbates the pedal edema of heart failure.

It is often challenging to differentiate restrictive cardiomyopathy from constrictive pericarditis and cardiac catheterization may be required for their distinction. The diagnosis of pericardial constriction is suggested if there is past history of tuberculosis, cardiac surgery or radiotherapy. Also, the X-ray chest shows linear pericardial calcification and ECHO may reveal pericardial thickening with multiple parallel lines, casting a bright reflection. Computed tomography (CT) or magnetic resonance imaging (MRI) may be required to demonstrate pericardiac thickening. Moreover, in constrictive pericarditis, the cardiac chamber size, myocardial thickness, valve structure and ejection fraction are all normal (Table 13.2). Clinically speaking, constrictive pericarditis presents with sole or predominant right heart failure while restrictive cardiomyopathy often presents with biventricular failure.

Table 13.2: Differences between constrictive pericarditis and restrictive cardiomyopathy		
	Constrictive pericarditis	**Restrictive cardiomyopathy**
Pericardium	Thick	Normal
Myocardium	Normal	Thick
Ventricles	Normal	Obliterated
Atria	Normal	Dilated
LV function	Normal	Mildly impaired
MV and TV	Normal	Regurgitation
MV inflow	Abrupt halt	Slow relaxation

MANAGEMENT ISSUES

Diuretics reduce dyspnea and edema and they are the mainstay of the medical management of restrictive cardiomyopathy. However, vigorous diuresis should be avoided since it would compromise ventricular filling, reduce cardiac output and even cause syncope. It is crucial to maintain sinus rhythm and to cardiovert atrial fibrillation by electrical (DC shock) or pharmacological (amiodarone) means. This is because atrial fibrillation leads to loss of atrial contribution to ventricular filling and shortens the diastolic filling time. Digoxin is best avoided for rate control and heart failure treatment, due to the high risk of ventricular arrhythmias in the presence of myocardial disease. Beta blockers and verapamil improve diastolic dystunction and control tachyarrhythmias. Specific therapies for restrictive cardiomyopathy are steroids for sarcoidosis and scleroderma as well as iron chelation therapy with desferrioxamine for hemochromatosis.

RECENT ADVANCES

The diagnosis of cardiac amyloidosis can now be confirmed by tissue biopsy. Amyloid shows birefringence when stained with Congo red and viewed under polarized light. Biopsy material can be obtained either from abdominal fat pad or from rectal and gingival sites. Endomyocardial biopsy is only performed if the above tissue biopsies are inconclusive and yet the clinical suspicion is strong.

Of late, cardiac MRI imaging with gadolinium enhancement has shown high sensitivity and specificity for amyloidosis. Recently, chemotherapy targeted against clonal plasma cells, that produce monoclonal light chains, has been tried as a treatment modality in cardiac amyloidosis. Also, sequential cardiac and stem cell transplant has been optimistically attempted.

CASE
14

Hypertrophic Cardiomyopathy

CASE PRESENTATION

A 48-year old man was brought to the emergency room by his office colleagues, because he had fainted while climbing stairs. There was no history of tonic-clonic jerks, frothing at the mouth or tongue bite. On regaining consciousness, the patient admitted having had two such episodes in the past, one while playing cricket with his son and the other while changing a flat-tyre of his car. There was no sensation of palpitation before these syncopal episodes. There was no past history of exertional chest pain or breathlessness, although at times he did feel light-headed at the end of the day. He did not suffer from hypertension or diabetes but he did smoke occasionally and took alcohol over the weekends. His father had passed away due to sudden cardiac death at the age of 42 and one of his elder cousin brothers was on treatment for heart disease.

On examination, the patient was not tachypneic and there was no sweating. The pulse rate was 88 beats/min. and regular, but two distinct peaks were felt in systole. Vigorous pulsations were seen over the carotid arteries. The BP was 118/78 mm Hg in the right arm. There was no anemia, cyanosis or sign of congestive heart failure. The apex beat was forceful and normal in location but two separate impulses were felt on palpation. The S_1 and S_2 were normal with a prominent S_4 audible in late diastole. A short systolic murmur was appreciated at the upper left sternal border that peaked in mid-systole and ended abruptly. There was no ejection click or palpable thrill and the murmur did not radiate to the neck. The lung fields were clear.

CLINICAL DISCUSSION

From the history and physical examination, this patient had syncope due to left ventricular outflow tract (LVOT) obstruction. The cause of obstruction possibly had a familial basis. ECG showed tall R waves with T wave inversion, in the lateral precordial leads, but there was no S-T segment shift or presence of Q waves. The rhythm was sinus and the Q-T interval was not prolonged. The X-ray chest did not reveal any cardiomegaly or sign of pulmonary edema.

On ECHO, the left ventricle cavity was small in size with a normal ejection fraction. There was significant hypertrophy of the left ventricular walls, with hypertrophy of the interventricular septum (IVS) exceeding that of the LV posterior wall (LVPW). The anterior mitral leaflet (AML) impinged on the

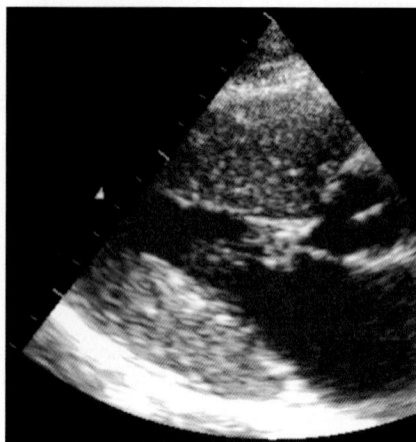

Figure 14.1: ECHO showing asymmetrical septal hypertrophy
impinging on the left ventricular outflow tract

hypertrophied septum during systole (Fig. 14.1). The aortic valve was structurally normal. On Doppler, an LV outflow tract gradient was demonstrated, proximal to the aortic valve. The high velocity jet had a typical concave appearance. On colour flow mapping, a mitral regurgitation jet was seen entering the left atrium. These ECHO findings are typical of hypertrophic obstructive cardiomyopathy (HOCM).

In retrospect, there were several pointers towards the diagnosis of HOCM, in the patient's history and physical examination. History of syncope with an ejection systolic murmur raised the possibility of aortic stenosis, but there was no ejection click, palpable thrill or radiation of murmur to the neck. Moreover on ECHO, the aortic valve leaflets were structurally normal and the outflow tract gradient was located proximal to the aortic valve. A positive family history of sudden cardiac death may be due to congenital channelopathies that cause ventricular tachyarrhythmias but the patient denied palpitation and the ECG showed sinus rhythm with a normal Q-T interval and no evidence of WPW syndrome. Moreover in most channelopathies, the heart is structurally normal. Atherosclerotic coronary artery disease is a prominent cause of premature sudden cardiac death which may run in families. However, coronary artery disease is rarely if ever associated with left ventricular hypertrophy, unless there is severe hypertension. Syncopal episodes are also uncommon, unless there is severe calcific aortic stenosis.

A double-peaked radial pulse that consists of a percussion wave and a tidal wave, is known as pulsus bisferiens. It indicates rapid early ejection of the left ventricle, followed by slow delayed emptying, after recoil of the vascular bed. Pulsus bisferiens is typical of HOCM but also occurs in combined aortic valve disease (stenosis plus regurgitation). The strong and bifid apex beat indicates forceful atrial contraction preceding ventricular systole. A prominent S_4 sound in presystole also carries the same significance. These are both clinical signs of reduced left ventricular compliance due to myocardial hypertrophy.

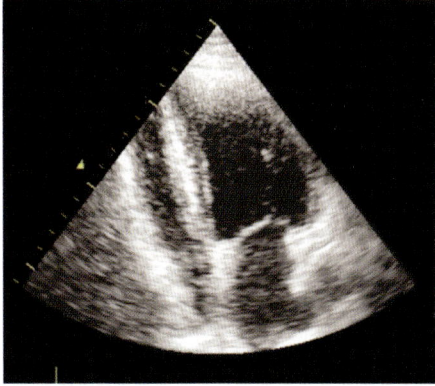

Figure 14.2: ECHO showing isolated hypertrophy
of the left ventricular apex

Hypertrophic cardiomyopathy is inherited as an autosomal dominant trait, caused by mutation of genes that encode for sarcomere proteins of the cardiac myocyte. It is characterized by left ventricular hypertrophy (LVH), systolic anterior motion (SAM) of the anterior mitral leaflet and dynamic left ventricular outflow tract obstruction (LVOTO). The left ventricular hypertrophy (LVH) is typically (but not exclusively) asymmetrical, involving the septum more than the free wall. Other causes of LVH such as severe aortic stenosis or uncontrolled hypertension are typically absent. This asymmetrical septal hypertrophy (ASH) superficially resembles the LVH observed in athletes. There is associated diastolic dysfunction of the left ventricle. In a specific variant known as apical cardiomyopathy, there is prominent hypertrophy of the ventricular apex without outflow obstruction (Fig. 14.2). The ECG typically shows deep inverted T waves in the precordial leads.

Systolic anterior motion (SAM) of anterior mitral leaflet (AML) is the hallmark of hypertrophic obstructive cardiomyopathy (HOCM). During later part of systole, the AML moves anteriorly to coapt with the IV septum (Fig. 14.3). This occurs due to drag or Venturi effect caused by high velocity in the LV outflow tract (LVOT). SAM occurs during late stage of systole when the LV cavity is smaller and causes dynamic LVOT obstruction. Therefore, the term hypertrophic obstructive cardiomyopathy (HOCM) is more appropriate. If no LVOT obstruction is demonstrable, the terminology used is non-obstructive idiopathic hypertrophic subaortic stenosis (IHSS).

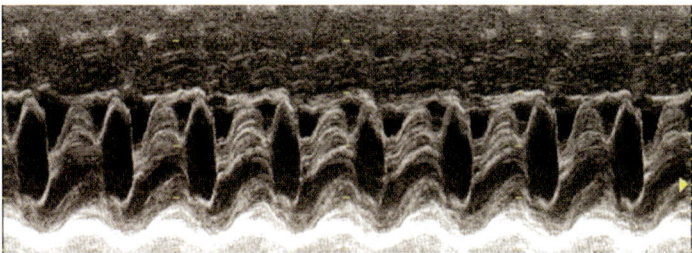

Figure 14.3: ECHO showing systolic anterior motion of anterior mitral leaflet

LVOT obstruction may be present at rest or become more pronounced after provocation. Provocation is provided by prolonged standing, Valsalva manoeuvre or giving sublingual nitrate. All these methods reduce left ventricular size and therefore increase the likelihood of LVOT obstruction. Conversely, squatting and isometric exercise such as hand-grip, increase left ventricular size and reduce the degree of LVOT obstruction.

MANAGEMENT ISSUES

The goals of treatment in hypertrophic cardiomyopathy are to control symptoms and to prevent sudden cardiac death (SCD). Symptoms include exertional dyspnea, typical or atypical angina, palpitations and syncope. Exertional symptoms are generally because of left ventricular hypertrophy with diastolic dysfunction and sometimes due to associated mitral regurgitation. Syncopal episodes are generally related to outflow tract obstruction and sometimes due to tachyarrhythmias. Patients should be advised to avoid strenuous exercise such as weight-lifting and not to participate in competitive sports.

Beta-blockers are the agents of first choice. They control heart rate, improve diastolic filling and reduce the outflow tract gradient. Calcium-channel blockers like verapamil are preferable, if beta-blockers are contraindicated. These agents are also used for rate-control if atrial fibrillation exists, although rhythm-control with amiodarone is preferable. This is because the loss of atrial contribution to ventricular filling, is often associated with clinical deterioration. All patients in atrial fibrillation should also receive an anticoagulant to reduce the risk of thromboembolism. Digitalis, diuretics and vasodilators should be avoided.

If the patient is symptomatic and refractory to medical treatment, surgical myomectomy is offered to relieve the outflow obstruction. In a patient who is at high-risk to undergo a surgical procedure, alcohol septal ablation can be performed by the percutaneous route. An injection of ethanol is given into one of the septal perforator branches to create an area of myocardial infarction and thereby widen the narrow outflow tract.

Sudden cardiac death (SCD) can be prevented by using an implantable cardioverter defibrillator (ICD), in selected high-risk candidates. These subjects are selected on the basis of identified risk factors for SCD. Risk factors include septal thickness >25 mm, outflow tract gradient >30 mm Hg, non-sustained ventricular tachycardia on 48 hour ambulatory Holter monitoring, history of recurrent syncope and atleast 1 SCD in a relative aged <45 years.

RECENT ADVANCES

Recently, cardiac magnetic resonance imaging (MRI) has been used to identify myocardial fibre disarray, as a risk factor for ventricular arrhythmias. Those subjects with this demonstrable abnormality should be candidates for implantable cardioverter defibrillator (ICD), to prevent sudden cardiac death (SCD). Alcohol septal ablation as an interventional strategy, has gained popularity.

15

Takotsubo Cardiomyopathy

CASE PRESENTATION

A 33-year old woman came on her own to the emergency room at 2 am, with the complaint of severe central chest pain and suffocation sensation, of one hour duration. She was also short of breath and sweating, but her chest pain did not radiate to the arms or lower jaw. There was no past history of exertional angina or dyspnea and she did not have diabetes or hypertension. There was also no history of a "flu-like" illness in the preceding week. She was pre-menopausal and her blood lipid profile had never been checked. She did not smoke, consume alcohol or abuse illicit drugs, although she was on antidepressant medications off and on. There was no history of premature coronary artery disease is any of her family members. Upon close questioning, the lady disclosed that she lived alone ever since her acrimonious divorce 3 months back, five years after a traumatic marriage.

On examination, the patient was of average built, anxious, sweating and tachypneic. The extremities were warm and her palms were moist. The pulse was rapid, fair in volume, at a rate of 110 beats/min. with a BP of 140/90 mm Hg. There was no anemia, cyanosis or pedal edema and the JVP was not raised. The thyroid gland was not enlarged and there was no tremor or eye-sign of thyrotoxicosis. The apex beat was normal in location and character and the precordium was unremarkable. The S_1 was loud and S_2 normal in intensity with a soft S_3 in early diastole. No murmur or friction rub was audible. There were few rales over the lower thirds of the lung fields.

CLINICAL DISCUSSION

From the history and physical examination, this patient developed acute left ventricular dysfunction preceded by severe chest pain. ECG showed sinus tachycardia and S-T segment elevation in practically all the leads, with upright T waves (Fig. 15.1). X-ray chest findings were borderline cardiomegaly and pulmonary interstitial edema but there was no mediastinal widening or pleural effusion. ECHO revealed a mildly dilated left ventricle with an ejection fraction of 35%. The distal septum and the left ventricular apex were hypokinetic (Fig. 15.2). The mitral and aortic valves were structurally normal and no colour flow jet or abnormal velocity was detected. No intracardiac mass or pericardial effusion was seen. The proximal aorta did not show dilatation or any sign of aortic dissection.

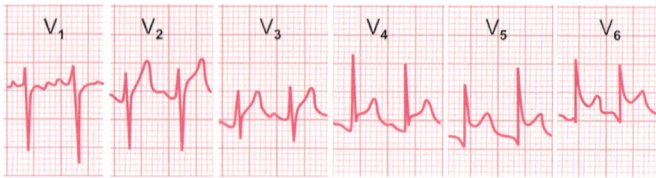

Figure 15.1: ECG showing sinus tachycardia with ST segment elevation

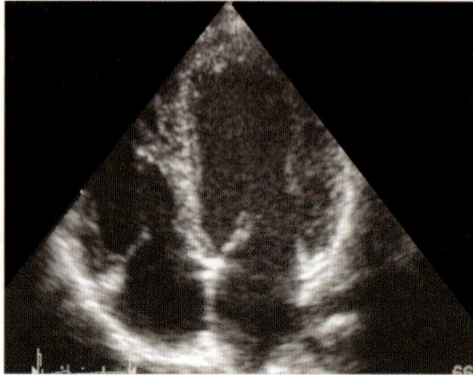

Figure 15.2: ECHO showing hypokinesia
of distal septum and apex

Whenever a patient has severe chest pain with S-T segment elevation on ECG and wall motion abnormality on ECHO, the first possibility to cross the mind is an acute coronary syndrome. This patient had no major coronary risk factors barring psycho-social stress, but her troponin-T test was positive. Since she came to a tertiary-care hospital, primary coronary angioplasty was planned. To everyone's surprise, the coronary angiogram turned out to be completely normal.

Another cause of severe chest pain with ECG findings is acute dissection of the aorta. These patients are usually hypertensive and develop acute aortic regurgitation with left ventricular volume overload. Our patient had no evidence of aortic root dilatation, cleavage of the aortic wall or aortic regurgitation. Rarely, dissection of the aorta can cause myocardial infarction, if the coronary ostia get occluded by the intimal flap.

Acute pericarditis also presents with chest pain and S-T segment elevation on the ECG. The pain is seldom excruciating and generally increases on deep inspiration. The troponin-T test is almost always negative. Presence of regional wall motion abnormality and reduced ejection fraction are unusual except if there is an additional component of myocarditis. Acute viral myocarditis is often preceded by a flu-like illness. It presents with acute left ventricular dysfunction but chest pain is unusual. Classical findings are global hypokinesia with depressed ejection fraction but regional wall motion abnormalities can occur if the myocardial inflammation is patchy in distribution.

Some other causes of acute left ventricular dysfunction also need to be considered. Low levels of serum electrolytes such as potassium, calcium and magnesium can impair myocardial contractility. Similarly, nutritional deficiency of vitamins and trace elements like thiamine, selenium and carnitine can also cause ventricular dysfunction. At times, thyroid storm and pheochromocytoma can present with left heart failure and should be ruled out by appropriate assays including serum thyroid hormone levels and urinary catecholamines. In our case, the left ventricular dysfunction was clearly related to psycho-social stress. Therefore, the definite diagnosis is stress-induced cardiomyopathy which is also termed as Takotsubo cardiomyopathy.

Table 15.1: Synonyms of Takotsubo cardiomyopathy
• Broken heart syndrome
• Stress induced cardiomyopathy
• Neurogenic myocardial stunning
• Transient ventricular apical ballooning

Takotsubo cardiomyopathy (Table 15.1) is a recently described entity also called the "broken heart syndrome", neurogenic myocardial stunning or transient left ventricular apical ballooning. Takotsubo is a Japanese name given to a round-bottomed narrow-necked fishing pot, used to trap an octopus. The shape of the left ventricle after apical ballooning, resembles this fishing pot. It occurs more often in postmenopausal, middle-aged women. Acute intense emotional stress is the usual triggering factor and the surge of catecholamines either causes microvascular vasospasm or direct myocyte injury. Additionally, release of free fatty acids by adrenalin induced lipolysis and hypokalemia due to an excess of cortisol, impair myocardial contractility.

These patients usually present with severe chest pain and clinical signs of left ventricular dysfunction. The ECG shows S-T segment elevation in multiple coronary artery territories and the biomarker of myocardial injury, the troponin-T test, is generally positive. The ECHO shows wall motion abnormality of the left ventricular apex which does not conform to any particular coronary artery territory and typically spares the basal segments. Coronary angiography does not show any major occlusive lesion in most patients.

MANAGEMENT ISSUES

Before the clinical profile of this entity was clearly elucidated, many women with Takotsubo cardiomyopathy were probably managed as anxiety related panic attack or menopausal syndrome. Some were thought to have acute viral myocarditis while still others improved on their own while being investigated for thyroid hyperfunction and pheochromocytoma. When the patients present with chest pain, S-T segment elevation and positive troponin-T test, it is prudent to manage them as acute coronary syndrome. Aspirin, clopidogrel, beta-blocker and low molecular weight heparin (LMWH) can all be instituted. An angiotensin converting enzyme (ACE) inhibitor with a diuretic can be added for heart failure management. Most patients make a rapid and event-free recovery, without any long-term disability or recurrence.

RECENT ADVANCES

Till a few years back, some stray case-reports of Takotsubo cardiomyopathy were published from Japan. With growing awareness about this entity, it is now being increasingly diagnosed across the globe. Recently carvedilol, a beta-blocker with additional alpha-blockade property, has been studied in a small cohort of cases and shown modest benefits.

Aortic Diseases

CASE

16

Aneurysm of Aorta

CASE PRESENTATION

A young man 21 years of age, came to his family physician with the complaint of progressively increasing shortness of breath of 2 months duration. There was no history of fever, productive cough, chest pain, hemoptysis or wheezing. The severity of his breathlessness had compelled him to discontinue basketball, his favorite sport. In fact he had been a regular member of his school and college basketball teams. Interestingly, he was inducted into his senior school team in class 8, when he was only 13 years of age, because of his extraordinary height. There was no history of nasal allergy, recurrent sore-throat, bronchial asthma or prolonged fever with joint pains during his childhood. He denied abusing tobacco, alcohol or any illicit drug. During a routine medical check-up before joining college 3 years back, he had been told of a heart murmur.

On examination, pulse was 88 beats/ min. regular, good in volume, with a BP of 160/70 mm Hg in the right arm. The JVP was not raised and there was no ankle edema. The precordium was hyperdynamic and there were visible pulsations in the aortic area. The apex beat was heaving in nature and located in the sixth intercostal space, in the anterior axillary line. A soft early diastolic murmur was audible along the left sternal border, accompanied by a S_3 sound in diastole.

The ECG was normal and X-ray chest showed mild cardiomegaly, with a hump over the upper right border of the heart. There was no sign of pulmonary congestion. ECHO revealed a dilated left ventricular cavity, with an end-systolic diameter of 52 mm and an ejection fraction of 45%. The aorta was enormously dilated, with a dimension of 68 mm between the leading edges of the anterior and posterior aortic walls. There was loss of the acute angle between the sinus of Valsalva and the ascending aorta. The aortic valve leaflets were not thickened, but appeared distant from the aortic walls. The mitral valve was structurally normal.

The patient was unusually tall, thin and lanky, with a height of 6 feet 1 inch and a body-weight of only 48kg. While examining the radial pulse, it was observed that his fingers were excessively long and tapering, with an extremely flexible wrist joint. Upon measurement, the distance between the finger-tips of the hands stretched sideways, was 6 feet 5 inches. In other words, the arm-span exceeded the height of the patient. Also, the pubis-to-heel length was more than the crown-to-pubis height. This physical appearance, coupled with the typical X-ray chest and ECHO findings of aortic root dilatation and aortic regurgitation, are highly suggestive of Marfan's syndrome.

CLINICAL DISCUSSION

The normal diameter of the aortic root in end-diastole, ranges from 20 to 37 mm. A dimension exceeding 40 mm constitutes aortic root dilatation, which has several causes (Table 16.1). If the dilatation is due to advanced age or systolic hypertension, the aortic annulus is normal in diameter. However, if the dilatation is caused by medial necrosis of the aortic wall or an inflammatory aortitis, the annulus is dilated with associated aortic regurgitation. In post-stenotic aortic dilatation, the aortic valve leaflets are thickened and calcific.

Table 16.1: Causes of aortic root dilatation	
• Atherosclerosis	Unfolded aorta Hypertension (elderly)
• Medial necrosis	Marfan syndrome Ehlers-Danlos syndrome
• Aortoarteritis	Syphilitic (rare) Takayasu disease
• Collagen disease	Reiter's syndrome Ankylosing spondylitis
• Post-stenotic	Aortic stenosis
• Post-traumatic	Aortic aneurysm

An aortic root diameter exceeding 60 mm, is a feature of aortic aneurysm which may be saccular or fusiform. The aneurysm appears as a balloon-like stretching of the aortic wall, which expands in systole and compresses the left atrium. The aortic valve cusps appear distant from the aortic walls, even when the valve is open in systole (Fig. 16.1).

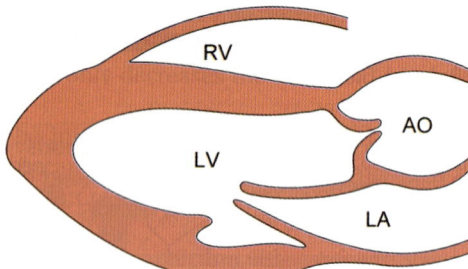

Figure 16.1: Diagram showing aneurysmal dilatation of the ascending aorta. RV: Right ventricle; LV: Left ventricle; AO: Aorta; LA: Left atrium

Marfan's syndrome is a connective tissue disorder, inherited as an autosomal dominant trait. The defect lies in the elastic fiber nature of the connective tissue. There is mutation in the gene encoding fibrillin-1, a connective tissue component and regulatory protein of transforming growth factor (TGF). Several striking abnormalities of the skeletal system are observed. The typical body habitus is a tall and slender figure with long tapering fingers and increased joint mobility. The pubis-to-heel measurement exceeds the crown-to-pubis length. Associated abnormalities include a high-arched palate, pectus carinatum, dislocated ocular lenses (ectopia lentis) and presence of inguinal hernias (Table 16.2).

Table 16.2: Clinical features of Marfan's syndrome		
Skeletal	**Cardiac**	**Others**
Tall stature	Aortic dilatation	Dislocation of lens
Joint hypermobility	Aortic aneurysm	High-arched palate
Arm-span > height	Aortic dissection	Crowded dentition
Long digits (arachnodactyly)	Aortic regurgitation	Pectus carinatum
Scoliosis and sternal deformity	Mitral valve prolapse	Inguinal hernia

Cardiovascular complications are initiated by cystic medial necrosis of the ascending aorta. There is dilatation of the aortic root with aortic valve insufficiency and left ventricular volume overload (Fig. 16.2). Catastrophic dissection involving the proximal aorta is a serious and potentially lethal complication. Mitral valve prolapse is sometimes associated.

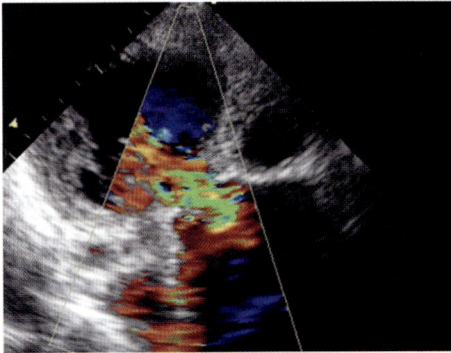

Figure 16.2: ECHO showing an aneurysmal aorta
with jet of aortic regurgitation

Although syphilitic aortitis is now distinctly rare, Takayasu's aorto-arteritis still afflicts young women in south Asia. It causes aneurysmal aortic dilatation and stenosis of the major branches emerging from the aorta. Blood pressure in the two arms may be different due to narrowing of subclavian artery on one side. On the other hand, hypertension may be present in the lower limbs due to reno-vascular stenosis. Therefore, Takayasu's aorto-arteritis is also designated as "reverse coarctation".

MANAGEMENT ISSUES

The medical management of an aortic aneurysm depends upon its size, the blood pressure and the presence or absence of aortic dissection. If the aneurysm is small, stable in size and there is no dissection, it suffices to adequately control the blood pressure. A drug with negative ionotropic effect such as a beta-blocker is preferable, since it reduces the shearing force on the aorta. The patient is counselled to avoid strenuous and burst activity like weight-lifting. Follow-up echo is recommended every 6 to 12 months, to assess the size of aneurysm and degree of aortic regurgitation.

Surgical intervention is considered if the aneurysm is growing in size on serial imaging, there is evidence of impending rupture or dissection, or if the aortic regurgitation is severe (Table 16.3). The affected segment of the ascending aorta is resected and replaced with a prosthetic graft.

Table 16.3: Indications for aortic aneurysm surgery
• Severe dilatation more than 50 mm
• Rapid aneurysm growth > 10 mm/year
• Dissection of the proximal aorta
• Severe aortic regurgitation

RECENT ADVANCES

Newer imaging techniques such as computed tomography (CT) and magnetic resonance imaging (MRI) have obviated the need for aortography, in the evaluation of aortic aneurysms. Serial imaging can identify an expanding size, impending rupture and an associated dissection.

17

Dissection of Aorta

CASE PRESENTATION

A 64-year old woman presented to the emergency department with sudden onset of severe chest pain, one hour back. The chest pain was central in location and it peaked instantly. The pain was also felt over the back between her scapulae, but did not radiate to the arms or neck. There was no history of suffocation, choking, palpitation or syncope and she had never experienced such chest pain before. She had a history of hypertension for which she had been prescribed multiple drugs. However, she was irregular with her medication and often skipped her doses. As a result, her BP hovered around 150/100 mm Hg on most occasions. She was not a diabetic but was advised to take atorvastatin for her elevated LDL-cholesterol. She did not consume alcohol, but smoked a pack of cigarettes per day for the last 40 years. Although distressed by severe chest pain, she managed to tell the attending doctor that the grip of her left hand felt weak since one hour.

On examination, she was clearly distressed but not dyspneic or diaphoretic. Pulse rate was 104 beats/min., with a BP of 174/106 mm Hg in her right arm. All peripheral pulses in the lower extremities were palpable, but a bruit was audible over the right carotid artery. The JVP was not raised and there was no pitting edema around the ankles. The apex beat was heaving in nature and slightly displaced outwards towards the axilla. The S_1 was normal and A_2 was loud, but there was no gallop sound. A faint early-diastolic murmur was audible along the left sternal border.

CLINICAL DISCUSSION

In an elderly patient, the most frequent but by no means the sole cause of excruciating chest pain is myocardial infarction. Other causes of severe chest pain are pulmonary embolism and spontaneous pneumothorax. The pain of pleuro-pericarditis, oesophagitis or costo-chondritis is seldom excruciating. Acute aortic dissection is an uncommon but potentially fatal cause of severe chest pain that merits a high index of clinical suspicion.

The ECG showed sinus tachycardia but no S-T segment shift and the troponin-T test was negative on admission. X-ray chest findings were mild cardiomegaly with a left ventricular contour and slight mediastinal widening due to aortic root dilatation. There was no basal atelactasis, pleural effusion or pneumothorax. ECHO revealed dilatation of the aortic root, with a false lumen cleaving the anterior aortic wall and having a blind end. An intimal flap separated the false lumen from the true aortic lumen (Fig. 17.1). On colour Doppler, a mosaic jet was observed in the left ventricular outflow tract, along the septum. There was no pericardial effusion. These findings were consistent with the diagnosis of acute dissection of the aorta.

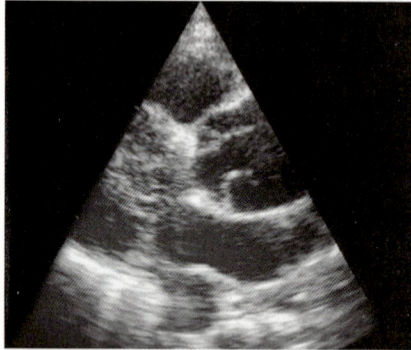

Figure 17.1: ECHO showing cleavage of the anterior aortic wall with intimal flap between true and false lumens

Acute myocardial infarction is an unlikely possibility in this case. The pain of myocardial infarction does not reach its maximum intensity instantly, but builds up gradually. Moreover, the radiation and accompaniments that are typical of the pain of myocardial infarction, were absent in this case. The ECG did not show S-T segment elevation and the troponin test was negative. On ECHO, cleavage of aortic wall and presence of aortic regurgitation are not typical features of acute myocardial infarction.

Table 17.1: Causes of aortic dissection
• Marfan's syndrome
• Coarctation of aorta
• Accelerated hypertension
• Hypertension in pregnancy
• Trauma; accidental or surgical

Dissection of aorta is often due to accelerated hypertension and may complicate hypertension in pregnancy. Other causes are aortic coarctation and Marfan's syndrome (Table 17.1). Aortic dissection cleaves the media of the aortic wall, with the adventitia and outer media forming the outer wall and the inner media and intima forming the inner wall. The false lumen produced by cleavage has a blind distal end while the proximal end communicates with the true lumen at the site of aortic tear. The intimal flap oscillates between the true and false lumens (Table 17.2). Other reasons for deformity of the anterior aortic wall are aortic root abscess in infective endocarditis and an aneurysm of the sinus of Valsalva.

Table 17.2: Typical features of aortic dissection

- Dilatation of the proximal aortic root > 42 mm
- Anterior or posterior wall thickness >15 mm
- Double echo-line of the involved aortic wall
- Space between outer and inner wall >5 mm
- False lumen within aortic wall with blind end
- Intimal flap between true and false lumens.

There are various classifications of aortic dissection. The simplest classification is of the Stanford group, which categorizes dissection as Type A (proximal), where the ascending aorta is involved and Type B (distal), where the ascending aorta is spared. This classification has prognostic as well as therapeutic implications. DeBakey Type I dissection extends from the ascending to descending aorta while Type II is confined to the ascending aorta. Type III is confined to the descending aorta and akin to Stanford Type B (Table 17.3).

Table 17.3: Classification of aortic dissection according to location

DeBakey type	Stanford group	Location of dissection	Incidence
I } II }	A	Ascending to descending aorta	10%
		Confined to ascending aorta	70%
III	B	Confined to descending aorta	20%

The complications of aortic dissection are related to the involvement of the aortic valve, pericardial sac and the arteries emerging from the aorta. Proximal involvement of the aortic valve can cause acute aortic regurgitation and heart failure. Hemorrhagic pericardial effusion can cause cardiac tamponade. Involvement of the coronary artery ostium can actually lead to myocardial infarction (Table 17.4). Involvement of the subclavian arteries can cause upper limb ischemia and discrepancy between the radial pulse volume on both sides. Involvement of carotid arteries can cause cerebral ischemia as in our case, who had weakness of the left hand and a right-sided carotid bruit. In distal aortic dissection, there may be mesenteric, renal, spinal cord or lower limb ischemia (Fig. 17.2).

Table 17.4: Atypical features of aortic dissection

- Occlusion of neck vessels
- Aortic valve regurgitation
- Left ventricular dysfunction
- Myocardial infarction
- Pericardial effusion

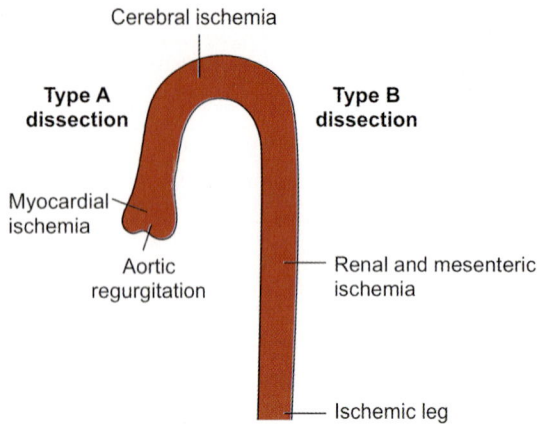

Figure 17.2: Complications of aortic dissection

MANAGEMENT ISSUES

The management of aortic dissection depends upon its location and extent, the presence or absence of complications and the hemodynamics of the patient. In distal (Type B) dissection, it generally suffices to control the blood pressure adequately. Agents with negative ionotropic effect such as a beta-blocker or verapamil are preferable as they reduce the shearing force on the aorta and the progression of dissection. A vasodilator such as sodium nitroprusside or an ACE-inhibitor may be added if the blood pressure remains significantly elevated. In the presence of abdominal, spinal or lower limb severe ischemia, an endovascular stent graft may be deployed to cover the dissection.

In proximal (Type A) dissection, surgical intervention is preferable unless the hemodynamics are compromised, in which case a conservative approach is adopted. The affected segment of the ascending aorta is resected and replaced with a prosthetic graft. The aortic valve and coronary ostia may need to be reconstructed. In extensive aortic dissection (DeBakey Type I), a combined approach that includes proximal resection with graft and distal endovascular stenting may be used.

RECENT ADVANCES

Newer imaging techniques such as computed tomographic (CT) angiography and magnetic resonance imaging (MRI) have obviated the need for aortography, in the evaluation of aortic dissection. The sensitivity and specificity of these tests, for a confirmatory diagnosis of aortic dissection, are in excess of 95%. The technique of percutaneous endovascular stenting to manage DeBakey Type I and III dissection, has also undergone considerable refinement.

18

Coarctation of Aorta

CASE PRESENTATION

A young man 27 years of age, presented to the out-patient clinic with general fatigue and difficulty in climbing even two flights of stairs. He was diagnosed to have systemic hypertension five years back and had been on antihypertensive drugs ever since. Besides his fatigue, he also complained of episodic headache with dizziness. These episodes were often related to undue physical exercise, emotional upset or to missing of his medication. There was no history of cyanotic spells or fleeting joint pains during childhood. He denied abusing tobacco, alcohol or illicit drugs.

On examination, there were no facial features of an endocrine disorder such as thyrotoxicosis, acromegaly or Cushing's syndrome, but his lower limbs were unusually thin. The radial pulse was 84 beats/min. and bounding in nature. The BP in his right arm was 170/100 mm Hg. Pulse amplitude over the femoral arteries was reduced in volume and delayed compared to the brachial pulsation. Also, there were visible pulsations in the suprasternal notch. The cardiac apex beat was heaving in nature and slightly displaced towards the left axilla. On auscultation, S_1 was normal, A_2 was loud and a presystolic S_4 was audible. An ejection systolic murmur was heard at the upper left parasternal area. Incidentally, the same murmur was also audible over the interscapular region. Soft continuous murmurs were also heard over the scapulae. On abdominal auscultation, there was no bruit heard over the renal arteries.

CLINICAL DISCUSSION

When confronted with a young patient with moderate to severe systemic hypertension, the clinician should be alert to the possibility of secondary hypertension. Incidentally, secondary hypertension constitutes less than 5% of all hypertensive patients, while most have primary or essential hypertension. Usual causes of secondary hypertension are:

- Endocrine disorders
- Renovascular disease
- Coarctation of aorta.

In this patient, ECG showed tall R waves in leads V_5 and V_6 with deep S waves in leads V_1 and V_2, indicating the presence of left ventricular hypertrophy (Fig. 18.1). X-ray showed mild cardiomegaly with a rounded contour of the left heart border. There was "notching" of the undersurface of the 4th to 8th ribs and

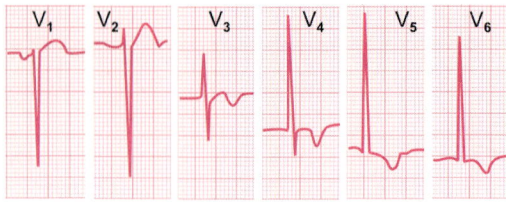

Figure 18.1: ECG showing tall R waves in V_5, V_6
with deep S waves in V_1, V_2

a "figure-of-3" appearance of the aortic arch. ECHO revealed concentric left ventricular hypertrophy with normal ejection fraction. Aortic valve was bicuspid with thickened leaflets and an insignificant gradient across the valve. The mitral valve was normal and there was no ventricular septal defect. Doppler signal from the suprasternal notch showed a pulsatile aortic arch with a distal aortic gradient that tapered into diastole. A mosaic jet was seen in the descending aorta, directed away from the transducer (Fig. 18.2).

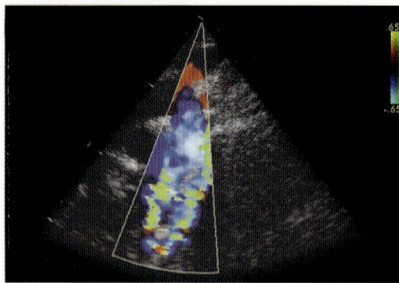

Figure 18.2: ECHO showing a mosaic jet
in the descending aorta

Coarctation of aorta is the most likely cause of hypertension in this case. There was clinical, radiological and cardiographic evidence of left ventricular hypertrophy. There were brachio-femoral delay, suprasternal pulsations, a parasternal and interscapular systolic murmur (coarctation itself) and continuous intercostal murmurs (collateral vessels). All these auscultatory findings are pathognomic of aortic coarctation. The murmur of coarctation itself may be continuous if the narrowing is severe, while presence of an ejection click indicates an associated bicuspid aortic valve. On X-ray chest, notching of the lower border of ribs indicates arterial collateralization, to by-pass the aortic obstruction. The "figure-of-3" appearance is produced by indentation of the aorta at the site of coarctation, with dilatation on either side of the narrowing. The suprasternal high velocity Doppler signal is characteristic of aortic coarctation.

Coarctation of the aorta is a localized narrowing of the aortic arch (Fig. 18.3), due to a fibrous ring encircling the wall or a shelf projecting into the lumen. The narrowing is in the region of the ligamentum arteriosum (juxta-ductal) and may be pre-ductal or post-ductal. The aorta distal to the narrowing is often dilated and aneurysmal. Coarctation may present in the neonatal period (infantile type)

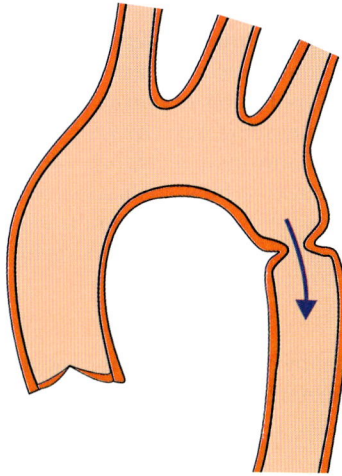

Figure 18.3: Coarctation of aorta

with heart failure, in which case the narrowing is diffuse, tubular and severe (hypoplastic aorta). In adult type coarctation, the narrowing is discrete, ring-like, less severe and detected during evaluation of systemic hypertension.

Some patients may complain of pain and/or weakness in the legs (claudication), due to reduced femoral blood flow. Brachio-femoral delay pertains to the difference in amplitude and timing between the brachial and femoral pulsations. Therefore, the blood pressure is higher in the upper limbs than in the lower limbs. If the left subclavian artery is also narrowed by coarctation, the blood pressure is only elevated in the right arm. In Takayasu's aorto-arteritis (pulseless disease), which is also called "reverse coarctation", the blood pressure is reduced in the upper limbs compared to the lower limbs, because there is stenosis at the origin of aortic arch branches.

Hypertension in coarctation of aorta is multifactorial. The aorta proximal to the narrowing is stiff and the carotid sinus baroreceptors are set at a higher level. Additionally there is a renal component, due to narrowing proximal to the renal arteries. Coarctation of aorta is associated with a bicuspid aortic valve in half the patients. Other cardiac anomalies are ventricular septal defect and mitral valve prolapse (Table 18.1). In 10 to 20% patients, there are intracranial aneurysms around the circle of Willis. Aortic coarctation may be associated with Turner's syndrome, characterized by a short-statured female with broad chest and a

Table 18.1: Abnormalities associated with coarctation
• Bicuspid aortic valve
• Mitral valve prolapse
• Ventricular septal defect
• Aneurysm sinus of Valsalva
• Intracranial Berry aneurysm

webbed neck. Long-term complications of coarctation are heart failure and stroke due to hypertension, dissection of proximal aorta and ruptured aneurysm of the sinus of Valsalva. The bicuspid aortic valve can develop stenosis or regurgitation and be the site of endocarditis. Finally, sub-arachnoid hemorrhage can occur due to ruptured intracranial aneurysm (Table 18.2).

Table 18.2: Complications associated with coarctation
• Congestive heart failure
• Endocarditis of aortic valve
• Dissection of proximal aorta
• Sub-arachnoid hemorrhage
• Stroke due to hypertension
• Aortic valve stenosis or regurgitation
• Ruptured sinus of Valsalva aneurysm

MANAGEMENT ISSUES

Management of secondary hypertension due to aortic coarctation, is governed by the same principles that apply to the treatment of essential hypertension. This involves the judicious use of a combination of antihypertensive agents. Several drugs are used including diuretics, beta-blockers, calcium-antagonists and ACE-inhibitors (or ARBs), since the hypertension is generally moderate to severe in grade and severity. Definitive treatment of aortic coarctation (systolic gradient > 30 mm Hg) is surgical excision of the area of aortic narrowing with an end-to-end anastomosis. A prosthetic tubular Dacron graft may also be interposed. Another technique is patch aortoplasty at the site of coarctation.

RECENT ADVANCES

Recently, the technique of percutaneous balloon aortoplasty has been developed. It is most suitable for discrete stenosis or if narrowing has recurred following surgical correction of coarctation. The incidence of restenosis after aortoplasty is reduced by stenting.

CASE

19

Sinus of Valsalva Aneurysm

CASE PRESENTATION

A 27-year old man was brought to the emergency room by his colleagues, with history of severe chest pain followed by light-headedness. The patient worked as a manual labourer in a construction company and his job involved strenuous activity, including lifting heavy weights. However, there was no past history of exertional chest pain or breathlessness. In fact, he had never suffered from any prolonged illness necessitating medication. He denied addiction to tobacco, alcohol or any other illicit drug. There was no past history of hypertension, diabetes, bronchial asthma or pulmonary tuberculosis. Moreover, none of his family members had heart disease or had succumbed to sudden cardiac death.

On examination, the patient looked anxious, but he was not in any distress. The hands were cold and clammy and the pulse was feeble in volume. The heart rate was 112 beats/min. with a BP of 96/64 mm Hg in the right arm, while lying in bed. There was no pallor, cyanosis or ankle edema and the JVP was not raised. The apex beat was normal in location and there was no parasternal heave. A continuous systolo-diastolic murmur was heard along the left sternal border, more so in the upper portion. The heart sounds could not be appreciated separately, because of the tachycardia as well as the long murmur. The breath sounds were vesicular in nature and air entry was normal and equal over both lung fields. There was no area of bronchial breathing or muffled breath sounds. No rhonchi, crepitations or pleural rub were audible.

CLINICAL DISCUSSION

From the history and physical examination, this previously healthy young man had severe chest pain, hypotension and a continuous murmur. ECG showed sinus tachycardia with narrow QRS complexes. There were no Q waves, S-T segment shift or T wave inversion. X-ray chest showed a normal sized heart. There was no basal atelectasis, pleural effusion or pneumothorax. The causes of severe chest pain with hypotension are:

- Myocardial infarction
- Pulmonary embolism
- Dissection of aorta
- Pneumothorax

In this case, acute myocardial infarction is unlikely because the patient had no coronary risk factors and the ECG did not show any Q waves or ST-T changes. Dissection of the aorta is also unusual in the absence of prior uncontrolled hypertension or coarctation of aorta. Spontaneous pneumothorax is a possibility, but this patient had no history of a predisposing lung condition such as bronchial asthma or pulmonary tuberculosis. Moreover, there was no clinical or radiological evidence of pneumothorax. Pulmonary embolism generally occurs after prolonged immobilization, but this patient was active and did not have any predisposing factor for deep vein thrombosis of the leg veins. Moreover, there was no area of collapse or consolidation on the chest X-ray.

On ECHO, all heart chambers were of normal size and all cardiac valves were structurally normal. There were no vegetations over the leaflets or any mass or thrombus in any chamber cavity. On careful examination of the short-axis view at the level of the aortic valve, a flow velocity and colour flow map was seen extending from the anterior aspect of aorta to the right ventricular outflow tract (RVOT). Therefore, the definite diagnosis in this case is ruptured aneurysm of the sinus of Valsalva.

An aneurysm of the sinus of Valsalva occurs as a result of congenital weakness of one of the sinuses, known as annulo-aortic ectasia. Rupture of the aneurysm may be spontaneous or due to increased aortic pressure, as occurs during isometric exercise. Sometimes the rupture may be due to the presence of infective endocarditis. Aneurysm of the noncoronary sinus ruptures into the right atrium, while that of the right coronary sinus ruptures into the right ventricle.

Table 19.1: Causes of continuous murmur
• Venous hum
• Mammary souffle
• Patent ductus arteriosus
• Aorto-pulmonary window
• Coarctation of the aorta
• Coronary arterio-venous fistula
• Ruptured aneurysm, sinus of Valsalva

In either case, there is continuous flow from the aorta to the right-sided chamber, since the aortic pressure is higher than the chamber pressure. This forms the basis of the continuous murmur heard when the aneurysm ruptures. There are several causes of a continuous murmur over the precordium (Table 19.1). Ruptured aneurysm of the left coronary sinus is the least common of all and may present with acute aortic regurgitation due to communication between the aorta and the left ventricle. Other causes of acute aortic regurgitation are chest wall trauma, infective endocarditis and dissection of aorta (Table 19.2).

Table 19.2: Causes of acute aortic regurgitation
• Dissection of aorta
• Annulo-aortic ectasia
• Infective endocarditis
• Blunt chest-wall trauma

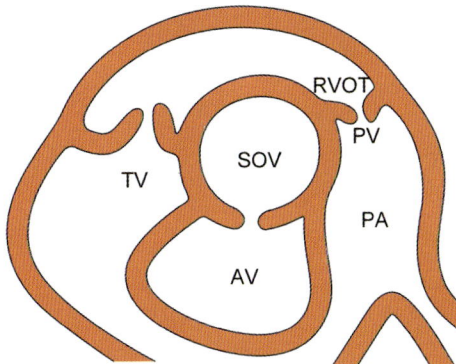

Figure 19.1: Diagram showing sinus of Valsalva aneurysm, anterior to the aortic valve. AV: Aortic valve; PA: Pulmonary artery; PV: Pulmonary valve; TV: Tricuspid valve; SOV: Sinus of valsalva; RVOT: Right ventricular outflow tract

An aneurysm of sinus of Valsalva (SOV) appears as an outpouching of the dilated coronary sinus anterior to the anterior aortic wall (Fig. 19.1), protruding into the right ventricular outflow tract (RVOT). A rupture of this aneurysm into the right ventricle produces right ventricular volume overload, of which there are several causes (Table 19.3). Aneurysm of sinus Valsalva or the fistula created by its rupture, is best visualized on transesophageal echocardiography (TEE). Cardiac abnormalities associated with a sinus of Valsalva aneurysm are bicuspid aortic valve and coarctation of aorta.

Table 19.3: Causes of right ventricular overload
• **From right atrium**
– atrial septal defect (ASD)
– tricuspid regurgitation (TR)
• **From pulmonary artery**
– pulmonary regurgitation (PR)
• **From left ventricle**
– ventricular septal defect (VSD)
• **From aortic root**
– ruptured aneurysm of sinus of Valsalva (SOV)

MANAGEMENT ISSUES

Newer imaging techniques such as computed tomography (CT) and magnetic resonance imaging (MRI) have obviated the need for root aortography, to evaluate the sinus of Valsalva. The size of the aneurysm, its precise location, the coronary sinus involved and the fistula created by its rupture, can be accurately visualized by these techniques. The management is surgical and involves resection of the aneurysm and the created fistula, repair of the aortic annulus and replacement of the affected segment with a prosthetic graft.

Pulmonary Diseases

20

Pulmonary Stenosis

CASE PRESENTATION

An 18- year old girl was taken to a neurologist by her parents. They had come back from a hill-resort vacation two days back, where she had fainted while playing badminton. There were no accompanying tonic-clonic movement, tongue-bite or frothing at the mouth. There was no past history of seizures, syncopal episodes, anoxic spells or squatting attacks during early childhood. A computed tomography (CT) scan of the brain and an electroencephalogram (EEG) were taken which were normal. The girl was referred to a cardiologist for evaluation of a heart murmur, which was detected by the astute neurologist.

On examination, pulse was of low volume at a rate of 84 beats/min. with a BP of 104/66 mm Hg. Prominent *a* waves were observed in the venous pulsations at the neck. The apex beat was normal in location and character. A sustained left parasternal heave was palpable, with the inner edge of the palm. The S_1 was normal and the S_2 appeared single; a right-sided S_4 was heard in diastole. A long and harsh ejection systolic murmur was audible over the upper left parasternal area. The murmur was not preceded by an ejection click or accompanied by a palpable thrill and it did not radiate towards the carotid arteries.

CLINICAL DISCUSSION

From the history and physical examination, this young girl probably had some cardiac outflow tract obstruction, which led onto syncope. The most likely diagnosis in this case is pulmonary valve stenosis (Fig. 20.1). The *a* waves in the jugular veins indicate forceful right atrial contraction against a noncompliant right ventricle. The parasternal heave is indicative of right ventricular hypertrophy. The S_2 appears single because the P_2 is muffled. If P_2 is audible, the splitting of S_2 is wide due to prolonged right ventricular (RV) ejection time. Other reasons for wide splitting of S_2 are right bundle branch block (delayed RV activation) and atrial septal defect (increased RV ejection volume).

The long and harsh ejection systolic murmur of pulmonary stenosis indicates turbulent flow across the narrow valve. Length and loudness of the murmur correlate with the severity of stenosis but once right ventricular failure sets in, the murmur becomes short and soft. The systolic murmur of pulmonary stenosis radiates towards the back and increases in intensity during inspiration.

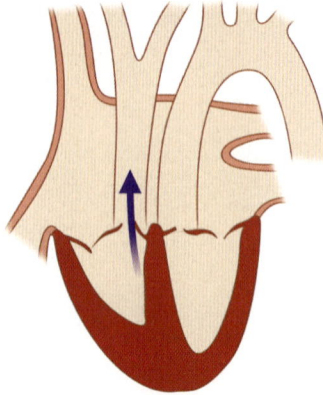

Figure 20.1: Pulmonary valve stenosis

An ejection click and palpable thrill are less often observed compared to aortic stenosis. Interestingly, the ejection click of pulmonary stenosis is the only right-sided heart sound that decreases during inspiration.

The ejection click marks the end of isovolumic contraction and heralds the onset of the ejection period. During inspiration, the increase in right ventricular end-diastolic pressure (RVEDP) leads to partial opening of the pulmonary valve and reduces the intensity of the ejection click. The ejection click is a feature of valvular stenosis and is not heard in infundibular stenosis. It also helps to differentiate pulmonary stenosis from atrial septal defect which produces a similar murmur with wide splitting of the second heart sound or S_2.

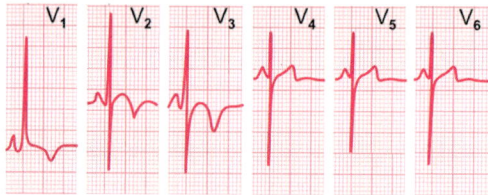

Figure 20.2: ECG showing tall R waves in V_1 to V_3, with inversion of T waves

ECG showed tall R waves in right precordial leads with T wave inversion (Fig. 20.2). There was right axis deviation of the QRS complex and right atrial enlargement (P. pulmonale). X-ray chest findings were an enlarged right ventricle to the right of midline, with a dilated pulmonary artery suggestive of post-stenotic dilatation. The lung fields were oligemic (Fig. 20.3). On ECHO, the left ventricle was normal in size with a normal ejection fraction and the free wall of the right ventricle was thickened. The mitral and aortic valves were structurally normal. The pulmonary valve leaflets were mildly thickened with mild systolic doming and restricted excursion. On colour flow mapping, a jet was observed in the proximal pulmonary artery, with increased systolic velocity across the valve on Doppler (Fig. 20.4).

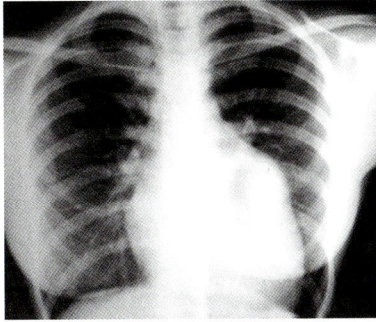

Figure 20.3: X-ray showing dilated pulmonary artery,
with oligemic lung fields

The ECG findings of right ventricular hypertophy (RVH) are tall R waves in lead V_1, S-T segment depression and T wave inversion (RV strain) and right axis deviation of the QRS vector. The voltage criteria of RVH are R in $V_1 > 4$ mm, R/S ratio in $V_1 > 1$ and S in $V_6 > 7$ mm. On chest X-ray, right ventricular enlargement and pulmonary artery dilatation are also seen in pulmonary hypertension but in that case there is pulmonary plethora and not oligemia. When pulmonary stenosis is a component of Fallot's tetralogy, the pulmonary artery is small (pulmonary atresia) and not dilated. In pulmonary hypertension, ECHO findings are a pulmonary regurgitant jet on color flow mapping and increased trans-tricuspid flow velocity (TR V_{max}).

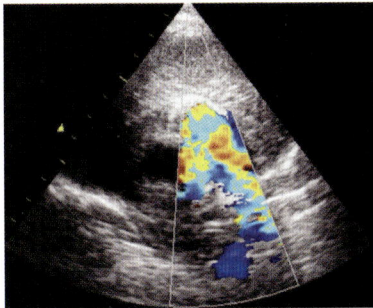

Figure 20.4: ECHO showing a color flow map
in proximal pulmonary artery

Pulmonary stenosis needs to be clinically differentiated from other conditions that produce a systolic murmur over the upper left parasternal area. These clinical entities are pulmonary hypertension, aortic stenosis and a high cardiac output state. Pulmonary hypertension is also associated with clinical, electrographic and radiological signs of right ventricular hypertrophy (Table 20.1) but the ejection murmur is accompanied by a loud P_2 sound and sometimes the murmur of pulmonary regurgitation. Moreover, the lung fields show pulmonary plethora and not oligemia.

The systolic murmur of aortic stenosis is often accompanied by an ejection click and a palpable thrill, radiates towards the neck and is better heard during

Table 20.1: Diagnostic criteria of right ventricular hypertrophy
- **Clinical:** Sustained left parasternal heave
- **ECG:** Tall R waves in right precordial leads
- **X-ray:** Cardiac silhouette to the right of midline
- **ECHO:** Thickening of right ventricular free wall

expiration. Moreover, there are clinical, electrographic and radiological signs of left ventricular hypertrophy. An innocent hemic murmur known as Still's murmur is sometimes heard in anemia, pregnancy, thyrotoxicosis and beri-beri disease. It is associated with a good volume pulse wide pulse-pressure and there is no ejection click or palpable thrill. On electrographic and radiological investigations, the cardiac chambers and valves are structurally normal.

Valvular pulmonary stenosis is often congenital in origin, as part of the Rubella syndrome. Rarely, valvular pulmonary stenosis is due to rheumatic heart disease (pulmonary valve involvement is least common) or carcinoid syndrome (tricuspid valve involvement is more common). Subvalvular or infundibular stenosis is often a part of Fallot's tetralogy. Supravalvular stenosis due to a discrete shelf-like band or a tunnel type deformity, is the least common form of pulmonary stenosis (Table 20.2).

Table 20.2: Causes of pulmonary stenosis

• **Congenital**	Rubella syndrome
• **Acquired**	Carcinoid syndrome
• **Subvalvular**	Fallot's tetralogy
• **Supravalvular**	Tunnel-type defect

MANAGEMENT ISSUES

There is no medical management of pulmonary stenosis. Surgery is indicated in the presence of symptoms, right ventricular hypertrophy and a systolic gradient above 50 mm Hg. The stenotic pulmonary valve has to be replaced by a surgical procedure, if the valve anatomy is distorted. Artificial pulmonary valve deployment is also feasible by the percutaneous route and expertise in this technique is growing. In isolated subvalvular or infundibular pulmonary stenosis, subvalvular muscle resection with valvotomy is the preferred procedure. When infundibular stenosis is part of Fallot's tetralogy, the procedure is combined with patch closure of the ventricular septal defect. Pulmonary regurgitation is the leading complication of valvotomy, which leads to dilatation of the tricuspid valve annulus and enlargement of the right-sided cardiac chambers.

RECENT ADVANCES

As mentioned above, expertise in the technique of percutaneous artificial pulmonary valve deployment has increased considerably. Also, percutaneous native valve balloon valvuloplasty has gained popularity in recent years.

Pulmonary Hypertension

CASE PRESENTATION

A 23-year old unmarried girl was brought to a physician with the complaints of progressively increasing breathlessness and fatigue on exertion, for the past 1 year. There was no history of fever, cough with purulent sputum, chest pain or hemoptysis. There was also no past history of seasonal allergy, bronchial asthma, anoxic spells or squatting attacks during her childhood. The patient had normal appetite without any weight-loss or history of night-sweats. On two occasions in the preceding month, she had fainted for less than five minutes. The fainting episodes were not preceded by palpitation, accompanied by tonic-clonic movements or followed by any abnormal behaviour. The parents of the girl denied any history of prolonged fever with painful joints, during her childhood or adolescence.

On examination, the pulse was feeble in volume at a rate of 92 beats/min. The BP was 106/68 mm Hg in the right arm and the patient was afebrile. A tinge of cyanosis was noticed over the tongue and lips but there was no clubbing of the finger-nails. Prominent *a* waves were observed in the venous pulsations at the neck, but there was no pedal edema. The apex beat of the heart was normal in position and had no special character. A parasternal heave was palpable along the left sternal border, with systolic pulsations felt over the 2nd left intercostal space. The S_1 was normal but the P_2 was accentuated. Splitting of S_2 could be appreciated upto the cardiac apex. No S_3 or S_4 gallop sound was heard. A high-pitched diastolic murmur was audible along the sternum. The breath sounds were vesicular in nature without any rhonchi or crepitations.

CLINICAL DISCUSSION

From the history and physical examination, this young girl probably had cardiac outflow tract obstruction, that was responsible for her dyspnea and fatigue and also led to syncope. The most likely cause of low cardiac output in this case is pulmonary arterial hypertension. The prominent *a* waves in the jugular veins indicate forceful right atrial contraction against a noncompliant right ventricle. A left parasternal heave indicates right ventricular enlargement while systolic pulsations over the pulmonary area are due to dilatation of the main pulmonary artery.

Accentuation of the P_2 is characteristic of pulmonary arterial hypertension. The fact that the P_2 is audible even at the cardiac apex is itself indicative of the fact that the P_2 is loud and the pulmonary hypertension is severe. Pulmonary hypertension causes pulmonary regurgitation even with a structurally normal pulmonary valve. This produces a high-pitched diastolic murmur known as the Grahm-Steel murmur. This murmur is short and does not increase during inspiration because the right ventricular end-diastolic pressure (RVEDP) is already high.

ECG showed tall R waves in right precordial leads and deep S waves in left precordial leads, indicative of right ventricular hypertrophy (Table 21.1).

Table 21.1: Criteria for right ventricular hypertrophy
• **Clinical:** Sustained left parasternal heave
• **ECG:** Tall R waves in right precordial leads
• **X-ray:** Cardiac silhouette to the right of midline
• **ECHO:** Thickening of right ventricular free wall

Tall P waves (P. pulmonale) were due to right atrial enlargement. X-ray chest findings were an enlarged right ventricle to the right of midline, with a dilated main pulmonary artery and normal pulmonary vasculature. On ECHO, the left ventricular size and ejection fraction were normal and the left atrium was not dilated. The mitral and aortic valves were structurally normal without any pressure gradient or abnormal jet on color flow mapping. There was no shunt across the interventricular septum.

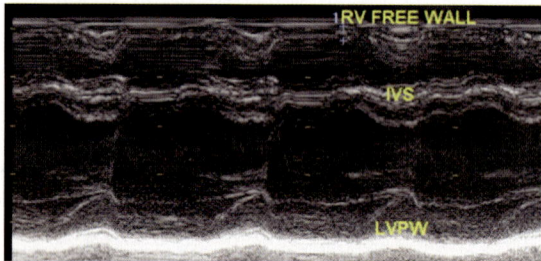

Figure 21.1: ECHO showing dilated right ventricle
with paradoxical septal motion

The right ventricle was enlarged and globular in shape. There was paradoxical motion of the interventricular septum, that moved away from the left ventricular cavity in systole (Fig. 21.1). On short-axis view, the dilated main pulmonary artery with its right and left branches, gave a "pair of trousers" appearance (Fig. 21.2). On color flow mapping, a pulmonary regurgitant jet was observed in the right ventricular outflow tract (RVOT). The pulmonary artery pressure, as estimated from the peak trans-tricuspid velocity (Vmax) by using the Bernoulli equation ($PG = 4\,Vmax^2$), was markedly elevated (Fig. 21.3).

RVSP = PAP;   RVSP – RAP = PG;   RVSP = PG + RAP; $RVSP = 4V^2 + RAP$

PG	:	Pressure Gradient
RAP	:	Right Atrial Pressure
PAP	:	Pulmonary Artery Pressure
RVSP	:	Right Ventricular Systolic Pressure

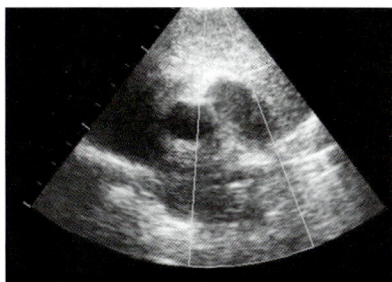

Figure 21.2: ECHO showing dilatation of
the main pulmonary artery

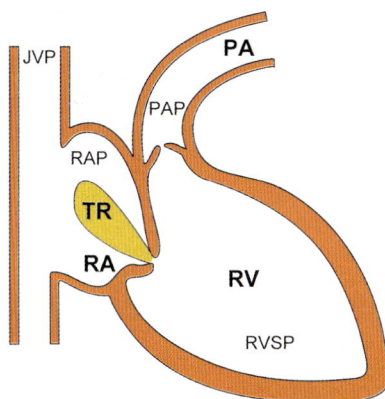

Figure 21.3: Estimation of pulmonary artery pressure from tricuspid regurgitant velocity
JVP: Jugular venous pressure; TR: Tricuspid regurgitation; RA: Right atrium;
RV: Right ventricle; PA: Pulmonary artery

The clinical, electrographic and imaging evidence of right ventricular enlargement with pulmonary artery dilatation is also present in pulmonary valve stenosis but with certain differences. In pulmonary hypertension, the P_2 is loud while in pulmonary stenosis, the P_2 is muffled. On chest X-ray, in pulmonary hypertension there is normal pulmonary vasculature or pulmonary plethora while in pulmonary stenosis, the lung fields may be oligemic. On ECHO, thickening of pulmonary valve leaflets with systolic doming and restricted excursion is a feature of pulmonary valve stenosis. On color flow mapping, in pulmonary hypertension, a regurgitant jet is seen in the right ventricular outflow tract. In pulmonary stenosis, a systolic jet is observed in the proximal pulmonary artery.

There are several causes of pulmonary hypertension (Table 21.2). Elevated left atrial pressure due to mitral valve disease (stenosis or regurgitation) is a prominent cause. However, in our patient the mitral valve was structurally normal, without any increased flow velocity or a regurgitant jet. Increased pulmonary blood flow due to a left-to-right shunt is another important cause. But in our case there was

Table 21.2: Causes of pulmonary hypertension
• **Increased pulmonary flow** Lt. to Rt. shunt; ASD, VSD, PDA
• **Raised left atrial pressure** Mitral valve disease; MS, MR
• **Chronic pulmonary disease** Chronic bronchitis, fibrosis
• **Obstruction to pulmonary flow** Thrombo-embolic, veno-occlusive
• **Primary pulmonary hypertension**

no ventricular septal defect or patent ductus arteriosus. Chronic obstructive or restrictive lung disease can also ultimately lead to pulmonary hypertension but there was no history of long-standing cough with expectoration or wheezing in our patient. Obstruction to pulmonary blood flow due to recurrent thromboembolism can also cause pulmonary hypertension but that is not the likely diagnosis in our case. Infrequent causes of pulmonary hypertension are intake of anorexigens, systemic sclerosis, sleep disordered breathing and HIV infection which are also unlikely possibilities in our patient. Therefore in all probability, our patient had idiopathic or primary pulmonary hypertension. The mild cyanosis could be due to minimal right-to-left shunting of blood across a patent foramen ovale.

MANAGEMENT ISSUES

In view of the pulmonary vasoconstriction and occlusion of the pulmonary vasculature associated with pulmonary hypertension, it is tempting to use vasodilators as therapeutic agents. Historically, a plethora of drugs have been used which include papaverine, nicotinic acid, isoxsuprine, cyclandelate and pentoxyphylline. However, none of them has withstood the test of time or found to be beneficial during evaluation in clinical trials. Among the established cardiovascular drugs, isosorbide nitrate, hydralazine, prazosin and verapamil have also been tried in the treatment of pulmonary hypertension but their benefits have been modest. Antiplatelet drugs such as low dose aspirin, clopidogrel and the newer agent cilostazol have also been used with mixed results. Phosphodiesterase (PDE) inhibitors such as sildenafil and tadalafil are the only agents with proven clinical benefit.

RECENT ADVANCES

Given the success of phosphodiesterase inhibitors in the treatment of pulmonary hypertension, recently two new classes of vasodilators have been added to the therapeutic armamentarium. The prostaglandin (PG) analogues epoprostenol and iloprost have proven vasodilatory action. The endothelin (ET-1) antagonist bosentan is the most promising out of the newer agents. It has a vasorelaxant as well as antiproliferative action.

22

Pulmonary Embolism

CASE PRESENTATION

A 72-year old elderly gentleman was rushed to the medical room of Toronto airport Canada, due to in-flight onset of severe chest pain, shortness of breath and profuse sweating. This happened minutes before the landing of his long-haul flight from New Delhi, India. He was a hypertensive on diuretic medication, but there was no past history of heart or lung disease. His son who received him at the airport, informed that the patient had undergone left knee replacement, six weeks prior to undertaking this journey.

On examination, the patient was restless, tachypneic, pale and diaphoretic. The pulse was rapid, irregular and feeble, at a rate of 110-120 beats/min. The BP in the right arm was 90/60 mm Hg. with a respiratory rate of 32/min and his temperature was 99.2⁰ F. The JVP was elevated and there was edema, erythema and tenderness over the left calf. The apex beat was normal in location and a parasternal lift was felt. There was tachycardia, loud P_2 and a right-sided S_3. No murmur or pericardial friction rub was audible. On chest auscultation, breath sounds were diminished over the base of the left lung posteriorly.

CLINICAL DISCUSSION

From the history and physical examination, the most probable diagnosis in this case is pulmonary embolism (PE) from deep vein thrombosis (DVT). ECG showed atrial fibrillation with fast ventricular response and T wave inversion in leads V_1 to V_3 (Fig. 22.1). There was no elevation of the S-T segment or presence of Q waves. X-ray chest findings were mild cardiomegaly, left basal atelectasis and a small left-sided pleural effusion (Fig. 22.2). There was no dilatation of the aortic root or widening of the mediastinum.

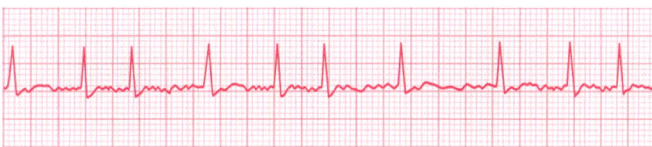

Figure 22.1: ECG showing atrial fibrillation with fast ventricular response

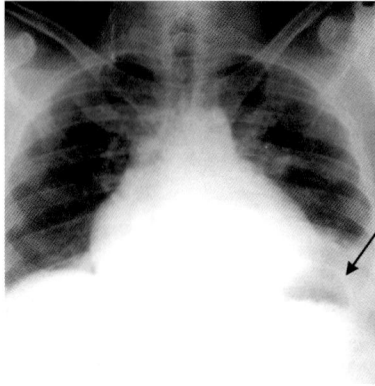

Figure 22.2: X-RAY showing left basal atelectasis
with small pleural effusion

ECHO revealed normal left ventricular size and ejection fraction, without any wall motion abnormality. There was a dilated and hypokinetic right ventricle with mild tricuspid regurgitation. The mitral and aortic valves showed some annular calcification, but there was no evidence of stenosis or regurgitation. There was no sign of aortic root dissection. There were also no vegetations on leaflets, ventricular thrombus or pericardial effusion.

There are several reasons for severe chest pain with dyspnea, sweating and hypotension. Acute myocardial infarction is the leading possibility, but the ECG did not show S-T segment elevation or presence of Q waves. Moreover, there was no regional wall motion abnormality of any left ventricular myocardial segment. Dissection of aorta may be considered, but there was no aortic root dilatation or cleavage of the aortic wall with a false lumen. Spontaneous pneumothorax generally occurs on a background of chronic lung disease with emphysema, but there was no such history in this patient. Moreover, there was no evidence of pneumothorax on the chest X-ray but only a small pleural effusion. Therefore, pulmonary embolism remains the strongest diagnostic possibility.

Pulmonary embolism is common and potentially life-threatening but often underdiagnosed clinical condition, associated with considerable morbidity and mortality. There is obstruction of pulmonary vasculature by a thrombus, fat, air or a tumour fragment. By and large, deep vein thrombosis (DVT) of the leg veins is the leading source. Predisposing factors are venous stasis, hypercoaguable state and injury to venous endothelium. Reasons for venous stasis are prolonged bed rest and immobility due to trauma, surgery, congestive heart failure or stroke. Long-distance air travel (economy-class syndrome) is also implicated. Hypercoaguability can be due to several reasons which may be inherited or acquired. Inherited defects are protein-C, protein-S or antithrombin-III deficiency and excess of homocysteine or fibrinogen. Acquired factors are estrogen therapy, malignancy, disseminated intravascular coagulation (DIVC) and antiphospholipid antibodies (APLA).

The clinical presentation of pulmonary embolism (PE) is extremely variable and is sometimes non-specific. Most patients present with pleuritic pain and dyspnea, with a variable degree of circulatory embarassment. In massive PE, there is hypotension and shock while in submassive PE, there is normotensive right ventricular dysfunction. Rarely, PE may present with insiduous onset of pulmonary hypertension. The clinical signs of acute PE are tachypnea and tachycardia, with or without hypotension. There is evidence of right ventricular strain in the form of elevated JVP, parasternal heave, loud P_2 and right-sided S_3. Signs of lower limb deep vein thrombosis (DVT) are edema, erythema and tenderness over the calf region.

PERTINENT INVESTIGATIONS

A large variety of investigations are performed for the diagnosis and assessment of pulmonary embolism. ECG invariably shows sinus tachycardia, sometimes with P. pulmonale, unless the patient is in atrial fibrillation. Right bundle branch block and T-wave inversion in leads V_1 to V_3 indicate right ventricular strain. The $S_1Q_3T_3$ pattern, although specific for pulmonary embolism (PE), is seen in a minority of patients (Table 22.1). On chest X-ray, there may be basal atelactasis

Table 22.1: ECG features of pulmonary embolism
• Sinus tachycardia (invariable)
• Atrial fibrillation (sometimes)
• P. pulmonale (in sinus rhythm)
• Right bundle branch block
• Rightward QRS axis deviation
• Dominant R wave in lead V_1
• T wave inversion in V_1 to V_3
• The $S_1 Q_3 T_3$ Pattern prominent S in L_I significant Q in L_{III} inverted T in L_{III}

and a small pleural effusion. Classical finding of pulmonary infarction is a wedge-shaped homogenous opacity above the diaphragm known as Hampton's hump or an oligemic lung segment which constitutes the Westermark's sign (Table 22.2). ECHO may reveal a dilated and hypokinetic right ventricle with mild tricuspid regurgitation and sometimes a right ventricular thrombus. Echocardiography is more often used to exclude other entities that mimic PE such as myocardial infarction, aortic dissection and pericardial tamponade.

Table 22.2: X-ray findings in pulmonary embolism
• Basal atelectasis
• Small pleural effusion
• Oligemic lung segment (Westermark's sign)
• Wedge-shaped opacity (Hampton's hump).

On arterial blood gas (ABG) analysis, hypoxemia is invariably present if the PE is massive. Hypocapnia and respiratory alkalosis also occur unless there is ventilatory limitation, in which case there is hypercapnia. D-dimer is a degradation product of cross-linked fibrin and its quantitative assay is used for the diagnosis of PE. However, it is more useful as a "rule-out" test, with a high negative predictive value. Duplex ultrasound is a combination of Doppler venous flow detection and real-time B-mode imaging. It plays a pivotal role in the diagnosis of lower extremity deep vein thrombosis (DVT). The most reliable finding of DVT is non-compressibility of a venous segment.

Ventilation-perfusion (V-Q) scanning used to be popular for the diagnosis of PE, prior to the advent of high-resolution contrast-enhanced computed tomography (CT). Its diagnostic accuracy is greater when it is clubbed with a clinical probability score than when used alone. Presently, it is reserved for those who cannot tolerate intravenous contrast because of allergy or renal failure. Contrast enhanced computed tomography (CT) is now considered the 'gold-standard' imaging modality for the diagnosis of PE. New generation CT scanners can visualize sixth-order branches of the pulmonary vasculature with high resolution. They have virtually replaced the older technique of invasive pulmonary angiography. Classical findings on CT are filling defect and abrupt cut-off of a vessel. Magnetic resonance (MR) pulmonary angiography can only detect large proximal PE and is not reliable for segmental and sub-segmental emboli.

MANAGEMENT ISSUES

The choice of therapy in pulmonary embolism is largely individualized and depends upon the clinical severity. Needless to say, hemodynamic and respiratory support are of paramount importance in those patients who present with shock or hypotension. Anticoagulants are the mainstay of treatment and should be initiated instantly pending investigations, to prevent further extension of an already formed thrombus. Sub-cutaneous low molecular weight heparin (LMWH) such as Enoxaparin is preferable, because of predictable dose response and no need for laboratory monitoring. The new-drug Fondaparinux, a factor Xa inhibitor can also be used. When unfractionated heparin is used, the international normalized ratio (INR) should be 1.5 to 2.5 times the control, for full therapeutic effect. Importantly, certain conditions in the differential diagnosis of PE, such as aortic dissection and pericardial tamponade, are contraindications to anticoagulation.

Thrombolytic therapy accelerates the lysis of acute pulmonary embolism, but is associated with an increased risk of major hemorrhage. It is reserved for massive PE, with hypotension and severe right ventricular dysfunction. If thrombolysis fails or is contraindicated, percutaneous embolectomy can be performed. However, it can only be used in the main arteries and if attempted in smaller branches, can cause perforation. Finally, if there is an absolute contraindication to anticoagulation or failure of the same and there is a proximal venous thrombus, an inferior vena caval (IVC) filter can be placed. It provides a screen to prevent lower limb or pelvic emboli from travelling to the lungs.

CASE
23

Obstructive Pulmonary Disease

CASE PRESENTATION

A 63-year old man visited a chest physician with the complaints of fever, breathlessness, cough and wheeze, for the past 1 week. The fever was of moderate grade, without chills, rigors or night-sweats, but was associated with body-ache and fatigue. He did feel breathless for the past several years, but his dyspnea had worsened since the onset of fever. He was orthopneic in bed but denied paroxysms of nocturnal dyspnea. The cough was associated with copious purulent sputum especially during morning hours, but there was no hemoptysis. The patient also experienced tightness in the chest on walking and he was aware of wheezing. His appetite was moderate and there was no history of significant weight loss. On specific questioning, he admitted smoking about 20 cigarettes daily, for the last over 35 years.

On examination, he was obviously dyspneic and orthopneic in bed and his accessory muscles of respiration were working. The face was puffy and hyperemic and there was mild cyanosis over the tongue and lips. The extremities were warm and sweaty. Clubbing of the finger-nails was noticed and there was edema over the ankles. The JVP was raised, trachea was central and there were no palpable lymph nodes in the neck. The pulse rate was 104 beats/min with a good volume that decreased appreciably during inspiration. The BP was 136/84 mm Hg, temperature 101.6^0 F and the respiratory rate was 28 per minute.

The antero-posterior diameter of the chest was increased, giving it the shape of a barrel. The percussion note over both lung fields was hyper-resonant and the upper border of the liver was percussed in the 6th right intercostal space. Bilateral expiratory rhonchi with scattered crepts were audible over the entire lung fields, with normal air-entry. The cardiac apex beat could not be located but there was a palpable parasternal heave. The S_1 was normal with a loud P_2. A soft early-diastolic murmur followed the P_2. A pansystolic murmur was also audible over the lower left parasternal area, that did not radiate towards the axilla. On abdominal examination, the liver edge was palpable 5 cm below the costal margin and was pulsatile. There was no other organomegaly or sign of free fluid in the abdominal cavity.

CLINICAL DISCUSSION

From the history and physical examination, the most likely diagnosis in this case is chronic obstructive pulmonary disease (COPD). The fever with worsening dyspnea and purulence of sputum indicates acute exacerbation of COPD, which is not uncommon among smokers. There were signs of respiratory distress (working accessory muscles), polycythemia (facial hyperemia), deoxygenation (cyanosis) and chronic lung suppuration (finger-nail clubbing). The raised JVP, enlarged liver and ankle edema indicate right heart failure which, when it is due to COPD, is known as corpulmonale. An appreciable decline in pulse volume during inspiration, is termed as pulsus paradoxus. Besides COPD, other causes of pulsus paradoxus are status asthmaticus and constrictive pericarditis.

A barrel-shaped chest with hyper-resonance over the lung fields and a "pushed-down" liver are indicative of hyperinflation, which is termed as pulmonary emphysema. Because of hyperinflated lungs, the cardiac apex beat is difficult to locate. In acute exacerbation of COPD, the adventitious breath sounds (rhonchi and crepts) are audible over the entire lung fields and the air-entry is equal. A parasternal heave with a loud P_2 and an early-diastolic murmur of pulmonary regurgitation are indicative of pulmonary arterial hypertension. Pulmonary hypertension leads to secondary tricuspid regurgitation which produces a lower parasternal pansystolic murmur and an enlarged liver which is sometimes pulsatile. The neck veins are distended with a prominent *y* descent.

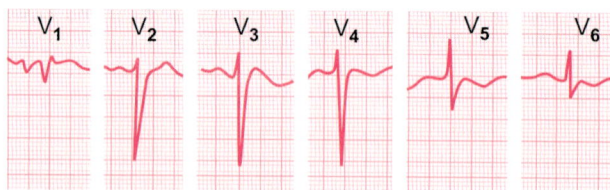

Figure 23.1: ECG showing non-progression of R wave
in the left precordial leads

The ECG shows low voltage of the QRS complexes, with non-progression of the R wave in precordial leads from V_1 to V_6 (Fig. 23.1). Due to clock-wise rotation of the heart, the right ventricle underlies most of the precordium, producing a rS pattern in most precordial leads. Other ECG features are tall R waves in right precordial leads (right ventricular hypertrophy), tall P waves (right atrial enlargement) and rightward deviation of the QRS vector (Table 23.1). The cardiac

Table 23.1: ECG abnormalities in COPD
• Low voltage QRS complexes (rS pattern)
• Right ventricular hypertrophy (tall R in V_1)
• Right atrial enlargement (P. pulmonale)
• Right axis deviation of QRS vector (RAD)
• Atrial tachyarrhythmias e.g. fibrillation (AF)

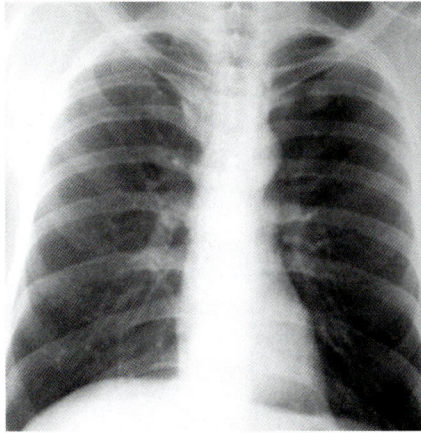

Figure 23.2: X-ray showing a tubular heart
with hyperlucent lung-fields

rhythm can be sinus tachycardia, atrial fibrillation or even multifocal atrial tachycardia.

The chest X-ray shows a tubular-shaped heart which appears small because of hyperinflation of the lungs (Fig. 23.2). The main pulmonary artery is often dilated. The lung fields are hyperlucent with prominent broncho-vascular markings. Due to hyperinflation, the intercostal spaces are wide and the domes of the diaphragm are flat and pushed downwards (Table 23.2).

Table 23.2: X-ray chest findings in COPD
• Tubular heart
• Hyperinflated lungs
• Dilated pulmonary artery
• Wide intercostal spaces
• Flat domes of diaphragm

Transthoracic ECHO is sometimes difficult to perform in patients of chronic obstructive lung disease, because of a poor acoustic window due to emphysema. Nevertheless, ECHO may reveal a dilated right ventricle that loses its triangular shape and becomes more globular. There is paradoxical motion of the interventricular septum, that moves away from the left ventricular cavity in systole. On short-axis view, the dilated main pulmonary artery with its right and left branches, gives a "pair of trousers" appearance (Fig. 23.3). On colour flow mapping, a pulmonary regurgitation (PR) jet may be observed in the right ventricular outflow tract (RVOT). The pulmonary artery pressure, estimated from the tricuspid regurgitant velociy, is elevated.

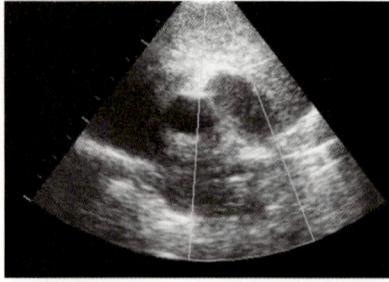

Figure 23.3: ECHO showing dilatation of main pulmonary artery

PERTINENT INVESTIGATIONS

Besides an ECG, X-ray and ECHO, other pertinent investigations in COPD are hematological, biochemical and bacteriological. The hemoglobin is high due to polycythemia while the leucocyte count is elevated with predominant neutrophils, because of the bacterial infection. The ESR is also increased because of chronic pulmonary suppuration but if very high, should alert us to the possibility of pulmonary tuberculosis. Blood glucose and liver and kidney function tests are done to rule out diabetes mellitus and other organ dysfunction. The sputum is examined by Gram staining to identify the causative organism. Sputum is also microscopically examined for acid fast bacilli (AFB) and fungal hyphae. Appropriate cultures are performed to identify suitable antimicrobial therapy. For patients in respiratory distress, arterial blood gas (ABG) analysis is done which may show hypoxemia, hypercapnia and respiratory acidosis.

MANAGEMENT ISSUES

The treatment of acute exacerbation of COPD includes antibiotics to treat the infection and bronchodilators to relieve airway obstruction. The antibiotic choice may be empirical or based on sputum culture report. Bronchodilators are given systemically or by the inhalation route and include theophylline, salbutamol, ipratropium and corticosteroids. Supportive treatment includes antipyretics, expectorants and oxygen therapy. Among the cardiovascular drugs, calcium blockers like verapamil and diltiazem may be used to control the heart rate. Betablockers and digoxin are avoided because of the risk of bronchospasm and ventricular arrhythmias respectively. Pulmonary hypertension can be treated with the phosphodiesterase (PDE) inhibitor sildenafil, prostaglandin (PG) analogue epoprostenol or an endothelin (ET-1) receptor antagonist bosentan.

Pericardial Infections

CASE
24

Acute Pericarditis

CASE PRESENTATION

A 26-year old man presented to the emergency department, with a dull precordial chest pain of 12 hours duration. The chest pain was not associated with suffocation or choking sensation and did not radiate to the arms. But the pain worsened when the patient took a deep breath and it hurt to cough or sneeze. About five days back, he had a "flu-like" illness with low grade fever, aches and pains along with dry cough. There was no history of purulence in sputum, hemoptysis or wheeze. He smoked 5 cigarettes a day, consumed about a litre of beer over the week-end, but denied abusing any illicit drug. There was no history of premature coronary artery disease in his family. He also denied any history of sore-throat with joint pains during childhood and he had not undergone any recent dental or endoscopic procedure.

On examination, the patient was in obvious discomfort and preferred to sit up in bed and lean forward. The pulse rate was 110 beats/min. regular, with a BP of 110/70 mm Hg and the temperature was 100.6^0 F. At the neck, JVP was not raised, thyroid gland was normal and there were no palpable lymph nodes. There were also no erythematous areas, skin nodules, petechial spots or swollen joints. Throat examination revealed mild pharyngeal congestion, but there were no pustules over the tonsils. On inspection, the precordium was quiet and the apex beat normally located. Upon auscultation, a high-pitched scratchy sound was audible all over the precordium. The lung fields were clear without any rhonchi or crepts. The ECG showed sinus tachycardia and narrow QRS complexes, with elevation of the S-T segment in most leads (except aVR) and depression of the P-R segment (Fig. 24.1)

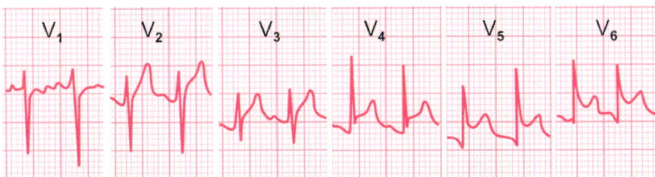

Figure 24.1: ECG showing sinus tachycardia with concave S-T elevation

CLINICAL DISCUSSION

When a patient presents with a short febrile illness, clinical signs of heart disease and some ECG abnormalities, possibilities that need to be considered are rheumatic fever, infective endocarditis, acute myocarditis and acute pericarditis. Rheumatic fever generally presents with a migratory polyarthritis, with or without cutaneous nodules or an evanescent skin rash. Infective endocarditis generally follows a dental or surgical procedure with a pre-existing valvular disease or a septal defect. Acute myocarditis is characterized by myocardial dysfunction and clinical signs of heart failure. Our patient presented with chest pain, had an audible pericardial rub and the ECG showed elevation of the S-T segment. Therefore, the most likely diagnosis in this case is acute pericarditis.

The chest pain of acute pericarditis is sharp in character and central in location. Therefore, it resembles the chest pain of myocardial infarction, but lacks the characteristic radiation and accompaniments of ischemic chest pain. The pain increases on deep breathing and coughing and therefore, patients prefer shallow respiration. The pain also worsens on lying supine and hence, the patient prefers to sit and lean forward.

The pericardial friction rub is a high-pitched, scratchy or squeaky sound, audible over the precordium along the lower left sternal border. It is better audible during inspiration, with the patient sitting up and leaning forward. Occasionally, the rub is accompanied by a palpable thrill, especially in patients with uremic pericarditis. The classical pericardial rub is triphasic and has three components, each related to a discrete phase of the cardiac cycle. Accordingly, there is a presystolic rub during atrial systole and a systolic and diastolic component related to ventricular systole and diastole respectively. Sometimes, the rub is a one-component or two-component sound, if there is associated atrial fibrillation or ventricular dysfunction. Sometimes the rub is evanescent and changes its quality on a day-to-day basis.

Table 24.1: Causes of S-T segment elevation
• Myocardial infarction
• Prinzmetal angina
• Ventricular aneurysm
• Dressler's syndrome
• Acute viral pericarditis
• Early repolarization variant

The most common and significant cause of S-T segment elevation on the ECG is coronary artery disease. S-T elevation occurs in acute myocardial infarction and in coronary vasospasm (Prinzmetal's angina). In patients with prior myocardial infarction, reasons for S-T segment elevation are Dressler's syndrome and ventricular aneurysm. S-T elevation also occurs in the early repolarization variant in which case the clinical profile is entirely normal (Table 24.1). The S-T

Table 24.2: ECG features of acute pericarditis
• S-T segment elevation is concave upwards
• S-T elevation is observed in nearly all leads
• T waves invert after S-T returns to base-line
• Q waves do not appear with ST-T changes
• R wave height is maintained in chest leads
• P-R segment is depressed in the limb leads
• Reciprocal S-T segment depression not seen
• Sinus tachycardia is almost invariably present
• Arrhythmias and conduction defects are unusual
• ECG changes do not evolve but resolve rapidly

segment elevation of acute pericarditis can be differentiated from that of acute myocardial infarction by several ECG features such as concave upward shape and concomitant depression of the P-R segment (Table 24.2).

PERTINENT INVESTIGATIONS

In patients with chest pain, the most frequently requested test after ECG is cardiac troponin-T. Troponin may be elevated in upto 50% of patients with acute pericarditis, thus limiting its diagnostic value. The total leucocyte count (TLC) and C-reactive protein (CRP) level may be elevated in acute pericarditis. A four-fold rise in antiviral antibody titre may occur, but is not diagnostic and often futile in the absence of specific antiviral therapy. Anti-streptolysin O (ASLO) titre and throat swab culture for beta-hemolytic Streptococcus are appropriate, if rheumatic fever is suspected. Suitable blood cultures are obtained, if the possibility of infective endocarditis is being entertained. In acute pericarditis, ECHO is useful to identify pericardial effusion and features suggestive of associated myocarditis. Usually, only a small rim of effusion is present and the left ventricular systolic function is normal. In myo-pericarditis, the ventricular function is mildly impaired but is generally reversible.

MANAGEMENT ISSUES

Treatment of acute pericarditis should first be targeted against a specific cause, if there is one. Examples include withdrawal of the offending drug in drug-induced pericarditis, hemadialysis for uremic pericarditis, thyroid hormone replacement for myxedema and suitable chemotherapy in malignant disease (Table 24.3). In most cases, non-steroidal anti-inflammatory drugs (NSAIDs) are first-line treatment, in the absence of a specific cause. In post-infarction Dressler's syndrome, aspirin is preferable over other NSAIDs. It is given in high-doses to begin with, to be tapered down over a period of time. Concomitant use of a proton pump inhibitor is recommended to reduce the risk of gastrointestinal bleeding.

Table 24.3: Causes of acute pericarditis
• Infective: viral, bacterial, tubercular
• Traumatic: accidental, cardiac surgery
• Malignant: metastasis, radiotherapy
• Autoimmune: rheumatoid arthritis, SLE
• Metabolic: uremia and myxedema
• Drug-induced: procainamide, hydrallizine
• Infarction: post-MI Dressler's syndrome

Colchicine may be used along with a NSAID in refractory and recurrent cases or alone if NSAIDs are contraindicated. Steroids should only be considered in the context of a systemic inflammatory disease. Steroids should not be used in bacterial or tubercular infection since they cause immunosuppression and in post-MI patients, as they interfere with scar formation. Pericardiocentesis and pericardectomy are rarely required in the treatment of acute pericarditis.

25

Pericardial Effusion

CASE PRESENTATION

A 66-year old gentleman visited the out-patient department of a tertiary-care hospital, with two months history of progressively worsening exertional breathlessness and increasing ankle swelling. There was no history of orthopnea or nocturnal dyspnea and he denied complaints of fever, productive cough, chest pain or hemoptysis. The patient was a known case of long-standing diabetes and hypertension. Recently, he was diagnosed to have chronic kidney disease and was advised peritoneal dialysis. His daily medication included lisinopril, frusemide, digoxin and glimepiride. There was no past history of angina pectoris or myocardial infarction, although he was told to have an "enlarged heart".

On examination, the patient was pale and mildly tachypneic, but not in any distress. The pulse was rapid, regular and low in volume, with an appreciable fall in pulse volume during inspiration. The pulse rate was 110 beats/min. with a BP of 104/66 mm Hg and respiratory rate of 24/min. The JVP was elevated without any noticeable descent during inspiration and there was pitting ankle edema. The precordium was silent and the apex beat was not visible but could be located only on palpation. On percussion, the area of cardiac dullness extended beyond the cardiac apex. The S_1 and S_2 were faintly audible on auscultation, but no murmur, gallop rhythm or friction rub was appreciated. Breath sounds were diminished over the left lung base posteriorly, with an area of bronchial breathing just above it. The rest of the lung fields were clear.

CLINICAL DISCUSSION

From the case history and particularly from the physical examination, the most likely diagnosis in this case is pericardial effusion. ECG showed sinus tachycardia with generalized low QRS voltages. The R wave amplitude varied on a beat-to-beat basis. X-ray chest findings were a markedly enlarged globular cardiac silhouette with a narrow basal vascular pedicle, giving the heart a "money-bag" appearance. The pulmonary broncho-vascular markings were normal. ECHO revealed a 2.5 cm wide echo-free space around the heart. There was noticeable collapse of the right atrium and right ventricle during diastole. The left ventricular function was normal.

In retrospect, there were several clinical pointers towards the diagnosis of pericardial effusion. A decline in pulse volume (fall in systolic BP>10 mm) during

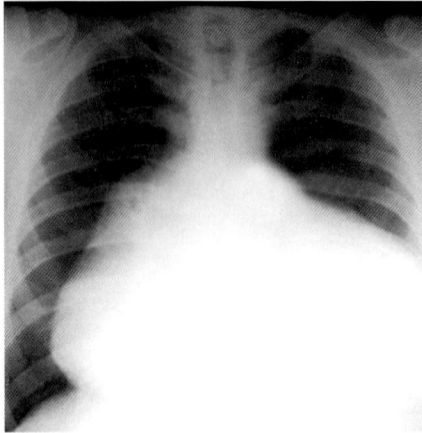

Figure 25.1: X-ray showing large cardiac silhouette with a narrow basal vascular pedicle

inspiration, is known as pulsus paradoxus. Increase in venous return shifts the interventricular septum towards the left ventricle, thereby reducing stroke volume. Besides pericardial effusion with cardiac tamponade, other reasons for pulsus paradoxus are constrictive pericarditis and status asthmaticus. A raised JVP without noticeable descent, indicates inadequate venous emptying during inspiration. Besides pericardial effusion, a raised and fixed JVP is a feature of superior vena caval obstruction.

A silent precordium with a non-palpable apex beat and muffled heart sounds indicate some intervening substance, may be fluid (pericardial effusion), air (pulmonary emphysema) or fat (morbid obesity). The combination of low BP, raised JVP and muffled heart sounds is known as Beck's triad and is characteristic of cardiac tamponade. The area of diminished breath sounds, dull percussion note and bronchial breathing just above it, indicate compression of the left lower lobe by the pericardial effusion. This constitutes the Ewart's sign.

On ECG, the beat-to-beat variability of QRS amplitude is known as electrical alternans. Its clinical counterpart is pulsus alternans. Total electrical alternans involves the QRS complex as well as the P and T waves. Besides cardiac tamponade, electrical alternans is also observed in severe left ventricular dysfunction. The "money-bag" heart, with enlarged cardiac silhouette and narrow vascular pedicle, is characteristic of pericardial effusion (Fig. 25.1). When cardiomegaly is due to heart failure, there is cephalization of pulmonary veins, along with hilar congestion, Kerley B lines and pulmonary edema.

Echocardiography is extremely valuable not only to confirm the presence of pericardial effusion (Fig. 25.2), but also to assess its magnitude and to identify signs of cardiac tamponade. It is also useful to exclude other causes of heart failure and to guide drainage of pericardial fluid. The quantity of pericardial fluid can be gauged from the width of the echo-free space around the heart (Table 25.1). The nature of pericardial fluid can be judged from careful analysis of the echo-free space. Transudative effusion is sonolucent while sanguinous fluid has high echodensity, sometimes with thrombus formation. Exudative effusion shows

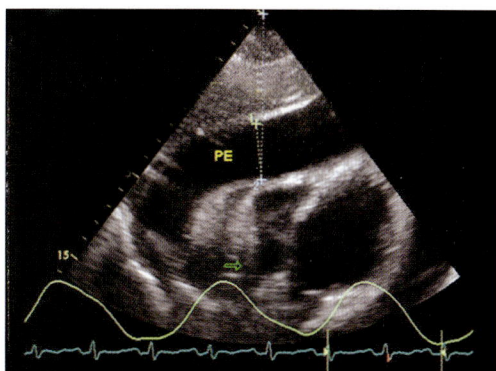

Figure 25.2: ECHO showing an echo-free space
all around the heart

Table 25.1: Quantification of pericardial effusion			
Amount	Volume	Posterior space	Anterior space
Small	< 100 ml	< 1 cm	—
Moderate	100-500 ml	1-2 cm	< 1 cm
Large	> 500 ml	> 2 cm	> 1 cm

fibrinous strands while malignant effusion may show echo-dense metastasis deforming the smooth pericardium.

A large pericardial effusion imposes constraint on filling of the cardiac chambers and hence impairs cardiac output. This serious clinical situation is known as cardiac tamponade. Tamponade results from a large volume of effusion, or rapid collection of a small effusion. A large effusion may accumulate gradually without causing tamponade, if the pericardial sac is compliant and gets adequate time to stretch itself. Therefore, rapidity of fluid accumulation is more important than absolute volume. The right-sided chambers are low-pressure structures and can easily get compressed by a large pericardial effusion. Right atrial collapse is a sensitive but less specific sign of cardiac tamponade. Right ventricular collapse, particularly if it lasts for more than one-third of diastole, is a less sensitive but more specific sign of cardiac tamponade.

Due to the constraint imposed by the effusion on the filling of the cardiac chambers, increased filling of the right ventricle (during inspiration) reduces filling of the left ventricle (hence cardiac output). Therefore during inspiration, tricuspid flow velocity increases while mitral flow velocity decreases. The converse occurs during expiration. A change in flow velocity exceeding 25% is considered to be diagnostic. This phenomenon of ventricular interdependence also forms the basis of pulsus paradoxus, which is observed clinically. This reciprocal relationship is also seen in constrictive pericarditis, where it is an important differentiating feature from restrictive cardiomyopathy.

Table 25.2: Causes of pericardial effusion		
• **Infective**	:	Tubercular pericarditis
• **Traumatic**	:	Accidental, surgical
• **Malignant**	:	Metastasis, irradiation
• **Metabolic**	:	Uremia, myxedema
• **Autoimmune**	:	Rheumatoid arthritis

There are several causes of pericardial effusion but inflammatory causes lead the list (Table 25.2). Tuberculosis is the commonest infection that causes pericardial effusion in the developing countries. Auto-immune disorders like rheumatoid arthritis and systemic lupus are also sometimes responsible for pericardial effusion. Idiopathic or viral pericarditis is usually associated with only a small effusion. Hemorrhagic effusion may follow accidental or surgical trauma or may be due to metastatic deposits in malignant disease. Metabolic disorders that cause pericardial effusion are uremia and myxedema (hypothyroidism).

PERTINENT INVESTIGATIONS

Pertinent investigations in pericardial effusion are completed blood count, tuberculin test, antinuclear antibodies, renal function tests and thyroid profile. The pericardial fluid is tested by cytology, bacterial culture and for adenosine deaminase activity and tumour markers when tuberculosis or malignancy are suspected.

MANAGEMENT ISSUES

Drainage of a large pericardial effusion by means of echo-guided (for safe needle entry) pericardiocentesis is the treatment of choice, particularly if there is cardiac tamponade. Most often the hemodynamic response to drainage is dramatic and gratifying. Fluid resuscitation may cause only transient improvement, but ionotropes has no role as cardiac contractility is not compromised. If there is no evidence of tamponade and the hemodynamics are stable, immediate drainage is unnecessary and the patient is managed conservatively. However, careful periodic assessment is mandatory. In tamponade due to aortic dissection, pericardiocentesis worsens hemodynamic stability and surgical drainage is preferable.

Antitubercular drugs are sometimes prescribed empirically if tubercular etiology is likely, or definitely if it is proven upon pericardial fluid analysis. Antinflammatory agents including steroids are employed for the treatment of auto-immune and inflammatory disorders. Malignant disease is treated with suitable chemotherapy or even radiotherapy which however, carries the risk of pericardial constriction.

CASE

26

Constrictive Pericarditis

CASE PRESENTATION

A 52-year old man visited the out-patient clinic of the department of internal medicine, with complaints of generalized fatigue, reduced appetite, increased abdominal girth and swelling over both ankles. He denied history of heavy alcohol intake, prolonged jaundice, hematemesis or altered bowel habits. About one year back, he was diagnosed to have pulmonary tuberculosis, for which he was prescribed anti-tubercular drugs for 6 months. But he was able to take his full medication only for 3 months, because he developed drug-induced hepatitis and therefore his rifampicin and isoniazid were stopped. However, he did take ethambutol and levofloxacin for the remaining 3 months. At present there were no complaints of fever, night-sweats, productive cough or hemoptysis. There was no history of diabetes, hypertension or heart disease in the patient or any of his family members.

On examination, the patient looked ill with a pinched face, thin emaciated arms, swelling around the ankles and a protuberant abdomen. He was not tachypneic or orthopneic and not in any form of distress. His conjunctiva and tongue were pale but there was no cyanosis or icterus. The pulse was fair in volume at a rate of 92 beats/min., with an appreciable fall in pulse volume during inspiration. The JVP was elevated 5 cm above the angle of Louis and it failed to fall appreciably during inspiration. The abdomen was distended, but there were no dilated veins or spider naevi on the skin surface. Shifting dullness was demonstrated, indicating free fluid in the abdominal cavity. The liver edge was palpable 8 cm below the right costal margin; it was slightly tender but not pulsatile. The precordium was silent and the apex beat was difficult to locate. There was no murmur or pericardial rub, but a high-pitched sound was audible in mid-diastole. There was some retraction of the apex of right lung on inspection, but both the lung fields were clear on auscultation.

CLINICAL DISCUSSION

From the history and physical examination, this patient definitely was in right heart failure. ECG showed sinus rhythm with low QRS voltages and non-specific T wave inversion. X-ray chest did not show any cardiomegaly, but there was a striking area of linear calcification along the left heart border (Fig. 26.1). There was fibrosis over the apical segment of the right lung. ECHO revealed normal size of all cardiac chambers, with normal left ventricular ejection fraction. There

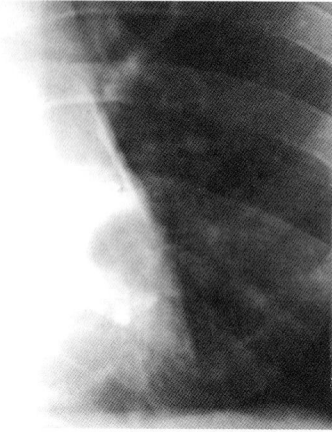

Figure 26.1: X-ray showing linear pericardial calcification

was no myocardial thickening or wall-motion abnormality and all cardiac valves were structurally normal. However, there was thickening of the pericardium, with multiple parallel echo-lines casting a bright reflection. Therefore, the most probable diagnosis in this case is constrictive pericarditis.

There were several typical clinical findings in this case. These were a variable pulse volume, raised JVP, silent precordium, no cardiac murmur and a sharp third heart sound in diastole. An appreciable decrease in pulse volume during quiet respiration is known as pulsus paradoxus. Besides constrictive pericarditis, pulsus paradoxus is observed in cardiac tamponade, chronic obstructive lung disease and status asthmaticus. A raised JVP that paradoxically rises even further during inspiration is known as Kussmaul's sign. Besides constrictive pericarditis, the Kussmaul's sign is observed in restrictive cardiomyopathy and after right ventricular infarction. The deep x descent on the JVP, represents the rapid phase of early diastolic ventricular filling. This is known as the "dip and plateau" pattern or the "square-root" sign of the ventricular pressure trace.

A silent precordium with a 'lost' apex-beat is a feature of pericardial effusion or constriction, morbid obesity and pulmonary emphysema. The third heart sound in constrictive pericarditis is the pericardial knock. It is a sharp and high-pitched sound, when compared to the classical S_3. The pericardial knock marks the termination of rapid early-diastolic phase of ventricular filling. Due to pericardial constriction, the inferior vena cava is dilated (Fig. 26.2) and there is congestive hepatomegaly. The spleen is also enlarged and ascites is present. These findings are picked up on clinical examination as well as by ultrasonography.

Constrictive pericarditis is a masquerader of several clinical conditions. Signs and symptoms are similar to those of congestive heart failure, but right-sided failure is more prominent and ascites is out of proportion to the degree of pedal edema. Hepatomegaly, ascites and edema may be misdiagnosed as cirrhosis of liver, if the neck veins are not observed carefully. Finally, if a patient is in atrial fibrillation, the diastolic knock may be misinterpreted as an opening snap and the diagnosis of mitral stenosis may be entertained.

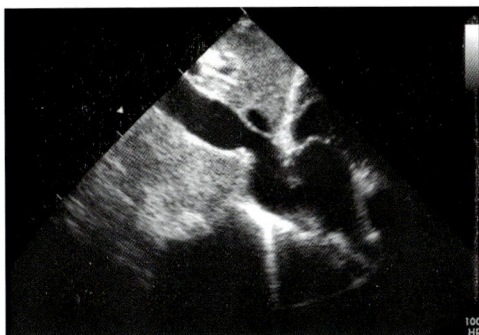

Figure 26.2: Abdominal ultrasound showing dilatation of the inferior vena cava

Table 26.1: Causes of constrictive pericarditis
• Tubercular pericarditis
• Bacterial pericarditis
• Cardiac surgery
• Chest irradiation

Constrictive pericarditis is most often preceded by a tubercular infection. Sometimes it may follow bacterial pericarditis but never viral pericarditis. Rheumatic pancarditis rarely causes constriction because the effusion is sero-fibrinous in nature and usually gets absorbed. Constrictive pericarditis may also follow chest irradiation or cardiac surgery (Table 26.1).

It is often difficult if not impossible to differentiate constrictive pericarditis from restrictive cardiomyopathy and cardiac catheterization may be required for their distinction. Restrictive cardiomyopathy is suggested by the presence of certain subtle echo features which are not observed in pericardial constriction. These features are small ventricles and large atria, thick mitral and tricuspid valve leaflets and mild impairment of left ventricular systolic function (Table 26.2).

Table 26.2: Differences between constrictive pericarditis and restrictive cardiomyopathy	Constrictive pericarditis	Restrictive cardiomyopathy
Pericardium	Thick	Normal
Myocardium	Normal	Thick
Ventricles	Normal	Obliterated
Atria	Normal	Dilated
LV function	Normal	Mildly impaired
MV and TV	Normal	Regurgitation

Moreover, the ventricular free walls may give a "granular-sparkling" appearance. Clinically speaking, restrictive cardiomyopathy generally presents with biventricular heart failure while constrictive pericarditis presents with sole or predominant right heart failure.

MANAGEMENT ISSUES

A two to three month period of conservative treatment can be tried in constrictive pericarditis, if the symptoms are mild. In the presence of signs indicating systemic venous congestion, it is naturally tempting to prescribe a diuretic to a patient of constrictive pericarditis. However, this approach is often counterproductive since ventricular filling declines further and cardiac output falls. Ionotropes like digoxin are unhelpful as there is no impairment of myocardial contractility. It is crucial to maintain sinus rhythm and to cardiovert atrial fibrillation by electrical or pharmacological means. This is because atrial fibrillation leads to loss of atrial contribution to ventricular filling and shortens the diastolic filling time. Pericardectomy by surgical means is the only effective treatment of constrictive pericarditis. It releases the ventricles from the restriction to diastolic filling, imposed by the rigid pericardial sac.

RECENT ADVANCES

The classical hemodynamic findings of constrictive pericarditis on cardiac catheterization not only helps to arrive at a definitive diagnosis but also help to differentiate between pericardial constriction and restrictive cardiomyopathy. These findings have been recently ellucidated. Due to the restriction imposed by the rigid pericardium on right ventricular filling, there is a sharp rise in early diastolic pressure followed by a flat pressure profile in mid and late diastole. This is reflected as a "dip and plateau" wave form on right ventricular pressure tracing and constitutes the "square-root sign". On inspection of the JVP, this pattern is observed as a prominent *x* descent.

Another hemodynamic finding is the reciprocal variation in the mitral and tricuspid inflow velocities with the phases of respiration, due to pericardial constraint. This reflects ventricular interdependence wherein right ventricular filling increases during inspiration at the expense of left ventricular filling. The converse happens during expiration when right ventricular filling decreases and left ventricular filling increases. This is reflected as an exaggerated (>25%) rise or fall of mitral and tricuspid inflow velocities, during inspiration and expiration.

Myocardial Infections

C A S E

27

Rheumatic Fever

CASE PRESENTATION

A 19-year old girl visited her family physician with the complaints of high-grade fever, pain in lower-limb joints and rash over the arms and legs, for the past 1 week. The fever started with pain in her throat and dry cough and was associated with chills but not rigors. There was no history of purulent sputum, chest pain, dyspnea, wheezing or hemoptysis. She also denied pain abdomen, vomiting, loose stools or burning sensation during micturition. The pain in her joints started in her right wrist and went on to affect both her ankles, which limited her walking ability. The skin rash was macular and erythematous, but there were no petechial spots or history of pruritus. The girl had not undergone dental extraction or any surgical procedure in the recent past. She did have sore-throat frequently during her childhood, but there was no history of anoxic spells or squatting attacks while playing.

On examination, the young girl looked ill, toxic and anxious. The pulse rate was 104 beats/min. with a BP of 104/66 mm Hg and her temperature was 100.6° F. Her extremities were warm and dry and there was no tremor or clubbing of the fingers. She was mildly anemic but not cyanosed or icteric. The erythematous rash over the extremities blanched on pressure. Her both ankles were mildly swollen and tender to touch, but there was no redness over the skin. On throat examination, there was mild pharyngeal congestion with enlarged tonsils that had few pustules. At the neck, the thyroid gland was not enlarged, JVP was not raised and there was no significant lymphadenopathy. The apex beat was normal in location and character and the precordium was quiet. The S_1 was soft and S_2 normally audible; no S_3 gallop or pericardial friction rub was appreciated. A low-pitched, mid-diastolic murmur was heard at the cardiac apex. The murmur was not preceded by an opening snap and did not undergo pre-systolic accentuation. The lung fields were clear without any rhonchi or rales.

CLINICAL DISCUSSION

From the history and physical examination, this young girl had a febrile illness with arthralgias, erythematous rash and a diastolic murmur. The obvious diagnosis with this constellation of clinical findings is acute rheumatic fever. The ECG showed sinus rhythm with a heart rate of 86 beats per minute and a

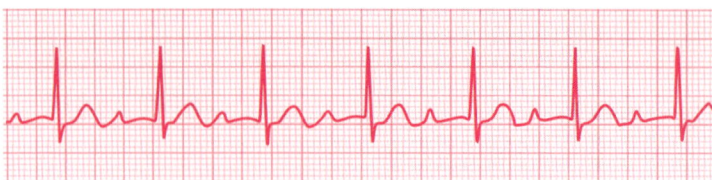

Figure 27.1: ECG showing prolongation of the P-R interval

prolonged P-R interval (Fig. 27.1). The QRS complexes were narrow and there was no S-T segment shift or T wave inversion. The X-ray chest did not show increased cardio-thoracic ratio or signs of pulmonary edema. ECHO revealed normal left ventricular size and systolic function, mild left atrial dilatation and a normal sized right ventricle. The mitral valve leaflets were mildly thickened (Fig. 27.2) with normal excursion and there was no diastolic doming of either leaflet.

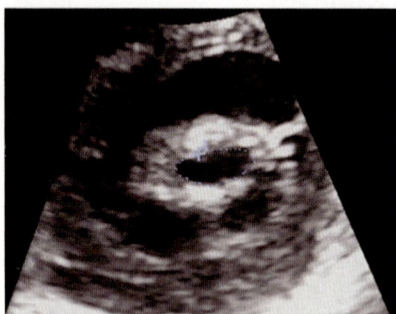

Figure 27.2: ECHO showing thickened
mitral valve leaflets

The hemoglobin was 10.4 g/dL with a leucocyte count of 11,800/cu.mm. of which 73% were neutrophils. The ESR was 55 mm in the 1st hour. Urine analysis showed traces of albumin but no WBCs or RBCs. The peripheral blood smear did not show any plasmodium parasite. The anti-streptolysin O (ASLO) titre was 366 IU with a C-reactive protein(CRP) value of 66 mg/L. Biochemical parameters including blood glucose, serum cholesterol and the renal and liver function tests were within normal limits. Urine and blood culture did not yield any bacterial growth. However, culture of the swab taken from the throat was positive for beta-hemolytic Streptococcus.

The clinical diagnosis of acute rheumatic fever is based on the presence of Jone's criteria (Table 27.1). Two major criteria or one major and two minor criteria, along with evidence of recent Streptococcal infection, are required to clinch the diagnosis. Major Jone's criteria are carditis, polyarthritis, chorea, erythema marginatum and subcutaneous nodules. Minor criteria are fever, arthralgia, history of rheumatic fever, elevated ESR, CRP and prolonged P-R interval. Evidence of a recent Streptococcal infection include positive throat swab culture and increased anti-Streptolysin O (ASLO) titer.

Table 27.1: Jone's criteria for the diagnosis of rheumatic fever		
Major criteria	**Minor criteria**	**Streptococcal infection**
• Carditis	• Fever	• History of scarlet fever
• Arthritis	• Arthralgia	• Throat swab culture + ve
• Chorea	• High ESR	• Streptococcal antigen + ve
• Eryth. marginatum	• Raised CRP	• High anti-Streptolysin O titre
• Subcut. nodules	• P-R interval	

A migratory or "fleeting" type of polyarthritis with fever and extreme weakness is the commonest manifestation of rheumatic fever. The arthritis typically involves the medium-sized joints such as the elbows, ankles and wrists. Chorea is usually observed in young children as an isolated entity, with rheumatic heart disease occuring a few days later. Erythema marginatum, which is hardly seen, is a pink rash on the trunk which blanches on pressure and is neither painful nor indurated. Rheumatic carditis is a pancarditis. Endocarditis manifests as a new murmur due to inflamed valve leaflets. Myocarditis presents as newly developed myocardial dysfunction. Evidence of pericarditis is a pericardial friction rub or presence of an effusion.

The major sequel of acute rheumatic fever is chronic valvular heart disease. Antibodies against streptococcal polysaccharide (carbohydrate cell wall) cross-react with cardiac tissues (myosin and laminin) to cause valve damage by molecular mimicry. During the acute stage, the mitral valve leaflets are inflamed resulting in a diastolic Carey-Coomb's murmur. Later on, due to smouldering disease, the valves are chronically damaged. Mitral stenosis, aortic regurgitation, mitral regurgitation and aortic stenosis, follow in that order of decreasing incidence.

MANAGEMENT ISSUES

The two pillars in the management of acute rheumatic fever are aspirin and penicillin. Aspirin can be given in a dose of 325 mg 4 times a day, during the stage of acute inflammation. The dose is gradually brought down, as the fever and pain subside. Care should be taken to co-prescribe a proton pump inhibitor like pantoprazole and to advise to take aspirin soon after a meal. If the patient is sensitive to aspirin, an alternative agent like ibuprofen or diclofenac may be used. Crystalline penicillin is administered in full doses parenterally, during the stage of acute inflammation. If the patient is hypersensitive to penicillin, a macrolide antibiotic such as erythromycin or azithromycin is chosen and the dose is 500 mg 6 hourly or 300 mg daily, respectively. Once the acute flare has settled down, long-term prophylaxis is suggested, particular to women, until they attain the age of 40 years. Antibiotic prophylaxis against infective endocarditis before a dental or surgical procedure, depends upon the nature and degree of chronic valvular involvement.

RECENT ADVANCES

As per the revised Jone's criteria for rheumatic activity in developing countries, erythema marginatum has been dropped as it is hardly ever seen. Polyarthralgia with raised ESR and high ASLO titre is no less common than objective arthritis and has been included as a major criteria.

Acute Myocarditis

CASE PRESENTATION

A 32-year old man presented to the emergency department with worsening breathlessness, over the preceding 3 days. Since the previous night, he was finding it difficult to lie flat in bed and had to sit up frequently to breathe. The patient was quite well until 5 days prior to his hospital visit, when he developed a "flu-like" illness. The low grade fever, headache, myalgia and mild sore throat had now settled down. There was no history of productive cough, chest pain or hemoptysis. There was also no history of skin rash, petechial spots or painful joints. He had not undergone any recent dental or endoscopic procedure. He did not suffer from recurrent pharyngo-tonsillitis during his childhood.

On examination, the patient was ill-looking and tachypneic. Pulse was fast and feeble and his extremities were sweaty. His heart rate was 116 beats/min with a BP of 104/68 mm Hg and the temperature was 98.8^0 F. There were no petechial hemorrhages under the finger-nails or in the conjunctiva and his joints were not swollen. The apex beat was displaced outwards and the S_1 and S_2 were normal. A soft S_3 was audible in early diastole, but there was no murmur. No pericardial friction rub was heard. There were few basilar rales over the lung fields.

CLINICAL DISCUSSION

From the history and physical examination, it is obvious that the patient had a short febrile illness, culminating in left ventricular dysfunction within a week. ECG showed sinus tachycardia, low QRS amplitude and non-specific T wave inversion. X-ray chest findings were enlarged cardiac silhouette, hilar congestion (Fig. 28.1), Kerley B lines and pulmonary edema. ECHO revealed a dilated left ventricle with global hypokinesia (Fig. 28.2). There was no abnormality of the cardiac valves, septal defect or presence of pericardial effusion.

When a patient presents with a febrile illness and ECG abnormalities, there are four main diagnostic possibilities. These are:
- Rheumatic fever
- Acute pericarditis
- Acute myocarditis
- Infective endocarditis.

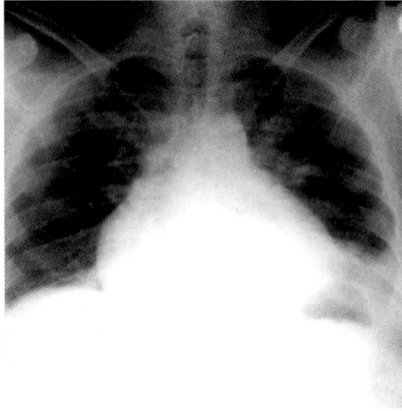

Figure 28.1: X-ray showing cardiomegaly with left pleural effusion

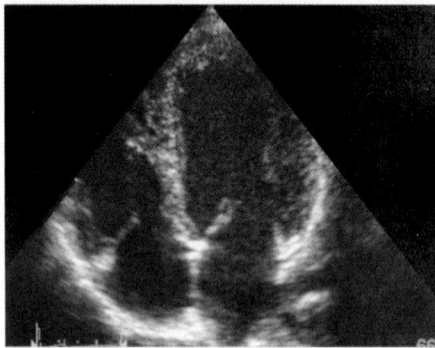

Figure 28.2: ECHO showing an enlarged globular left ventricle

Acute pericarditis is unlikely because the patient had no chest pain or S-T segment elevation on the ECG or pericardial friction rub on clinical examination. Moreover, left ventricular dysfunction is unusual in pericarditis, unless there is an associated component of myocarditis. Infective endocarditis is also unlikely because the ECHO did not show any abnormality of the cardiac valves or presence of a septal defect. Rheumatic fever is a pancarditis where myocardial dysfunction is accompanied by pericarditis (friction rub) and endocarditis (inflamed valve leaflets). Moreover, rheumatic fever generally presents with a migratory polyarthritis with or without cutaneous nodules and an evanescent skin rash. Therefore, the most probable diagnosis in this case is acute myocarditis.

Acute myocarditis is an inflammatory disease afflicting the heart muscle and causing myocardial dysfunction over a short period of time. Although global hypokinesia is the hallmark of myocarditis, regional wall motion abnormalities can occur, if myocardial inflammation is patchy in distribution. The myocardial damage and necrosis is immune-mediated and the cardiac troponin levels are often elevated. The etiology is most often viral and Coxsackie B virus or Echovirus

Table 28.1: Pathogens implicated in acute myocarditis	
• Viral	Coxsackie B, Echovirus, HIV
• Bacterial	C. diphtheriae, Mycoplasma
• Spirochetal	Lyme's disease, Leptospirosis
• Protozoal	Chaga's disease

are commonly implicated. Myocarditis may be bacterial as in Mycoplasma infection and Diphtheria. Rarely, it may be caused by a spirochete as in Leptospirosis or protozoa as in Chaga's disease (Table 28.1).

PERTINENT INVESTIGATIONS

The patient of acute myocarditis must be investigated to establish the inflammatory nature of the disease and the type of inflammation. The total leucocyte count (TLC), erythrocyte sedimentation rate (ESR) and C-reactive protein (CRP) helps to establish inflammation. Anti-streptolysin O (ASLO) titre and throat swab culture for beta-hemolytic Streptococcus are indicated, if rheumatic fever is suspected. Suitable blood cultures are obtained, if the possibility of infective endocarditis is being entertained.

Viral serology for the diagnosis of viral myocarditis is generally unhelpful, because the implicated viruses are ubiquitous in nature and antiviral drugs have no role in the treatment. Endomyocardial biopsy is rarely performed because of its low diagnostic yield, except in situations where a specific etiology is suspected on clinical grounds and needs to be confirmed on tissue analysis. These conditions are Loeffler's endocarditis, hemochromatosis and amyloidosis. Besides inflammation, electrolyte imbalance and nutritional deficiency are sometimes responsible for acute left ventricular dysfunction. These need to be excluded by appropriate tests such as serum potassium, calcium and magnesium levels. Thyroid hormone assay and urinary catecholamine levels are measured if thyrotoxicosis or pheochromocytoma are suspected.

MANAGEMENT ISSUES

The clinical features of myocarditis are similar to those of dilated cardiomyopathy, except that the onset of symptoms and signs is rapid. Therefore, the management of acute myocarditis is similar to that of dilated cardiomyopathy and follows the principles of standard heart failure treatment. The clinical manifestations not only evolve rapidly but also resolve within a short period of time. Loop diuretics are the mainstay of therapy to relieve pulmonary edema. An angiotensin converting enzyme (ACE) inhibitor or angiotensin receptor blocker (ARB) is added to reduce cardiac afterload and to improve ventricular performance. An aldosterone antagonist (spironolactone or eplerenone) may be added if symptoms persist on the above treatment. Digoxin has no role in the acute setting since atrial fibrillation is unusual. Antiviral drugs and immunomodulatory agents do not improve clinical outcomes.

RECENT ADVANCES

The role of auto-immunity in the pathophysiology of myocarditis and subsequent onset of dilated cardiomyopathy is being extensively investigated. However, so far neither anti-inflammatory drugs nor immunomodulatory therapy have been found to be successful. Auto-antibodies against beta-adrenergic receptors may also be relevant and patients who test positive for autoantibodies may respond more favourably to beta-blocker treatment.

Endocardial Infections

Aortic Valve Endocarditis

CASE PRESENTATION

A 64-year old gentleman presented to the hospital emergency service with fever for the past 3 days. The fever was high grade and associated with chills but there were no rigors. The patient was discharged 2 weeks back from this very hospital, having undergone an aortic valve replacement with a St. Jude's prosthesis for severe valve stenosis. Besides fever, he complained of headache, malaise, arthralgias and anorexia. He had not felt pain or noticed any redness at the sternal wound or at the site of intravenous cannula insertion. There was no history of productive cough, burning micturition, vomiting, pain abdomen or loose stools. He did not experience any significant chest pain or breathlessness. The patient denied having undergone any dental extraction or endoscopic procedure, after his surgery. He admitted having been noncompliant with the medication prescribed to him, at the time of discharge from the hospital.

On examination, he was ill-looking, toxic, febrile (101.8^0 F) and mildly tachypneic. Pulse was 110 beats/min with a BP of 130/60 mm Hg and his extremities were warm and sweaty. There was no sign of inflammation at the sternotomy wound or the site of intravenous line. The S_1 was loud, S_2 was sharp but no S_3 or S_4 was heard. There was an ejection systolic murmur along the left sternal border, but no pericardial friction rub was audible. Breath sounds were normal without any rhonchi or crepts. The abdomen was soft without hepato-splenomegaly or ascites. Additionally, there were petechiae under the finger nails (splinter hemorrhages) and sub-conjunctival spots (Roth spots) as well as tender nodules on the finger tips (Osler nodes).

The hemoglobin was 10.8 g/dL with a leucocyte count of 14,800/cu.mm; 86% were neutrophils and the ESR was 42 mm in 1st hour. Urine analysis showed albumin +1 with few RBCs but no WBC. ASLO titre was 180 IU with a CRP value of 48 mg/L. The biochemical parameters were Glucose 88 mg/dl, Creatinine 1.1 mg/dl, Bilirubin 2.2 mg/dl SGOT 24, SGPT 30 and Cholesterol 178 mg/dl. Urine culture did not yield any bacterial growth and throat swab culture was negative for beta-haemolytic Streptococcus. No pus was obtainable from the sternotomy wound for culture. Three sets of blood cultures were obtained, using aseptic skin precautions and all of them grew Staphylococcus epidermidis, after 72 hours of incubation.

ECG showed sinus tachycardia with few ventricular premature beats but there was no conduction block. The X-ray chest did not show any cardiomegaly, parenchymal lung lesion (pneumonitis) or mediastinal widening (mediastinitis). ECHO revealed normal left ventricular size and ejection fraction. There were irregular echo-reflective masses attached to the aortic valve leaflets with mild aortic regurgitation (Fig. 29.1).

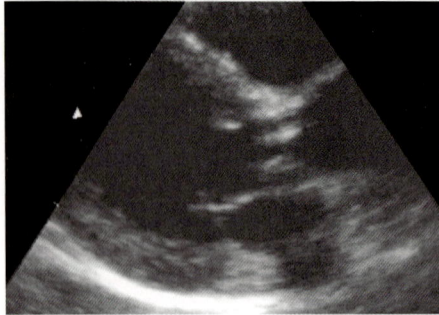

Figure 29.1: ECHO showing nodular masses
attached to aortic valve leaflets

Keeping in mind the history of a febrile illness with a prosthetic heart valve, positive blood cultures and demonstrable vegetations with aortic regurgitation, the most likely diagnosis in this case is aortic valve endocarditis.

CLINICAL DISCUSSION

Infective endocarditis may be caused by typical organisms, atypical bacteria and sometimes by fungi (Table 29.1). Non-infective endocarditis is observed in malignant disease (marantic), collagen disorder (Libman-Sacks) and rheumatic fever (pancarditis). High-risk lesions for endocarditis are regurgitant left-side valves (MR, AR), intracardiac shunts (VSD, PDA) and a prosthetic valve. Moderate-risk lesions are stenotic valves (MS, AS), MVP with MR and right-sided valves (TR and PS). Low-risk lesions are ASD, HOCM and MVP without MR. Modified Duke's criteria are popularly used for the diagnosis of endocarditis (Table 29.2). Fever is associated with various vascular and immunological phenomena. Blood cultures may be negative due to prior antibiotic therapy, fastidious or atypical pathogen and in case of fungal endocarditis. ECHO is used to detect vegetations, diagnose the underlying lesion, to look for complications and to evaluate the response to therapy. Transesophageal echocardiography (TEE) is a better approach for detecting complications, such as prosthetic valve dehiscence or aortic root abscess and for the timing of surgical intervention.

Table 29.1: Pathogens implicated in infective endocarditis		
BACTERIA	• Typical	Staphylococcus, Streptococcus
		HACEK * group bacteria
	• Fastidious	Legionella, Brucella
		Neisseria, Nocardia
	• Intracellular	Chlamydia, Coxiella
		Mycoplasma, Bartonella
FUNGI	• Typical	Candida, Aspergillus
*HACEK group: Haemophilus, Actinobacillus, Cardiobacterium, Eikenella, Kingella		

Table 29.2: Modified Duke's diagnostic criteria of infective endocarditis

Pathological criteria
• Micro-organism demonstrated by bacterial culture
• Active endocarditis on histological examination

Major criteria
• Positive blood cultures
• Typical organism consistent with endocarditis, on two separate blood cultures
• Organism consistent with endocarditis, from persistently positive blood culture
• Positive serology for Coxiella burnetti, Chlamydia psitacci or Mycoplasma

Evidence of endocardial involvement
• Prosthetic valve dehiscence, aortic root abscess, new valvular regurgitation

Minor criteria
• Predisposing heart condition e.g. prosthetic heart valve or intravenous drug use
• Fever more than 38^0C
• Vascular phenomenon (embolic complication, mycotic aneurysm, Janeway lesions)
• Immunological phenomenon (rheumatoid factor, nephritis, Osler's nodes, Roth spots)
• Microbiological evidence not meeting major criteria
• Echocardiographic changes not meeting major criteria

DEFINITE ENDOCARDITIS
• Pathological criteria plus 2 major, or 1 major and 3 minor, or 5 minor criteria

POSSIBLE ENDOCARDITIS
• 1 major and 1 minor, or 3 minor criteria

REJECTED DIAGNOSIS
• Firm alternative diagnosis
• Does not meet above criteria
• Resolution within 4 days of antibiotic therapy

MANAGEMENT ISSUES

The mainstay of the effective treatment of infective endocarditis (barring fungal endocarditis) is antibacterial drugs. Bactericidal drugs with low minimum inhibitory concentrations (MIC_{90}) against the identified organism are chosen. The intravenous route of administration is preferable to achieve high serum levels of the drug. This ensures adequate penetration of the antibiotic, since the vegetations are rich in necrotic tissue debris and therefore resist entry of the drug. A combination of 3rd generation cephalosporin with an aminoglycoside may be initiated, even when culture reports are pending, and are generally effective against Streptococcal endocarditis. Infection caused by Staphylococcus aureus is treated with flucloxacillin or vancomycin along with gentamycin or amikacin. Usually 2 to 4 weeks of treatment suffices in native valve Streptococcal infection while 6 weeks are required to treat Staphylococcal prosthetic valve endocarditis. The indications for surgical intervention in endocarditis are prosthetic valve dehiscence, aortic root abscess, fistula formation, refractory heart failure and recurrent embolic events (Table 29.3).

Table 29.3: Indications for surgery in endocarditis
• Fungal or resistant organism causing endocarditis
• Prosthetic valve dehiscence or aortic root abscess
• Heart block (septal abscess) or a fistula formation
• Valve regurgitation leading to refractory heart failure
• Recurrent systemic emboli despite adequate therapy

RECENT ADVANCES

The clinical spectrum of infective endocarditis has undergone a major change in the last two decades, for several reasons. Prevalence of Staphylococcal infection has increased with the widespread use of catheters, venous lines and pacing leads and the rising incidence of intravenous drug abuse. An entirely new HACEK group of bacteria has been identified as also a range of intracellular bacteria that can cause endocarditis. With the growing number of valve replacements, prosthetic valve endocarditis is on the rise. Finally, immunocompromised hosts such as HIV-infected patients and organ transplant recipients on immunosuppressive drugs are more likely to be infected by fungal organisms.

Tricuspid Valve Endocarditis

CASE PRESENTATION

A 32-year old male came to the out-patient department of a charitable hospital, with history of fever for the last 3 weeks. The fever was high-grade and associated with chills and night sweats, but there were no rigors. He also felt fatigued and had lost his appetite, leading to significant weight loss. However, he was not aware of his exact past body-weight. He also had cough with scanty mucoid sputum for one month, but there was no history of burning micturition, vomiting, pain abdomen or passing loose stools. There was also no history of dyspnea, chest pain or hemoptysis. The patient was unmarried and he was not accompanied by any attendant. He was a college drop-out, presently not engaged in any gainful employment. He admitted smoking and taking alcohol as well as drug-snorts, whenever he could afford them. He also sometimes abused intravenous illicit drugs.

On examination, the patient was emaciated, ill-looking, confused and febrile. The pulse rate was 110 beats/min. with a BP of 96/70 mm Hg and a temperature of 101.6^{0}F. He was mildly anemic but not cyanosed or icteric and there was pitting edema over the ankles. The neck veins were engorged and showed rapid y descent. There were multiple needle-prick marks over the veins on his forearms. On cardiac auscultation, a pansystolic murmur was heard over the lower left parasternal area; no gallop sound was audible. There were scattered rhonchi and crepts over the lung fields. On examination of the abdomen, there was hepatomegaly. The liver edge was palpable 5 cm below the costal margin and it was pulsatile. There was no splenomegaly or ascites.

PERTINENT INVESTIGATIONS

The hemoglobin was 9.2 g/dL with a total leucocyte count of 13,600/cumm. of which 78% were neutrophils; the ESR was 64 mm in the 1st hour. Urine analysis showed albumin +1 with 2-3 WBCs and 8-10 RBCs per high power field. ASLO titre was 110 IU with a CRP value of 62 mg/L. The biochemical parameters were Glucose 78 mg/dl, Creatinine 1.4 mg/dl, Bilirubin 1.8mg/dl, SGOT 79 and SGPT 53 and Cholesterol 144 mg/dl. The hepatitis B surface antigen was negative but his HIV-status was unknown. Urine culture did not yield any bacterial growth. Throat swab culture was negative for beta-hemolytic Streptococcus. Three sets

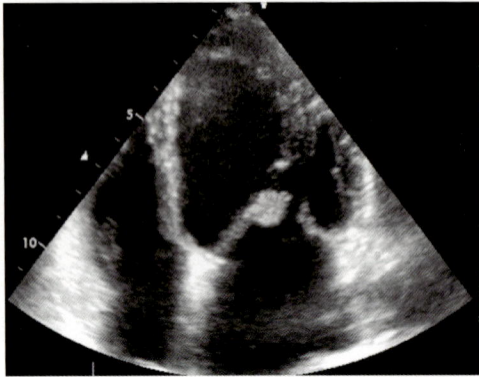

Figure 30.1: ECHO showing a nodular mass
attached to valve leaflet

of blood cultures were obtained, including from the veins of the forearms that bore needle-prick marks. Two out of the three cultures grew coagulase negative Staphylococcus aureus. One of the cultures grew Candida albicans.

ECG showed sinus tachycardia with narrow QRS complexes and no ST-T changes. X-ray chest did not show any cardiomegaly, but the broncho-vascular markings were prominent over both lung fields. ECHO revealed normal left ventricular size and ejection fraction. The mitral and aortic valves were normal. An irregular echo-reflective mass was observed, which appeared to arise from the tricuspid valve (Fig. 30.1). There was moderate degree of tricuspid regurgitation. Keeping in mind the history of a prolonged febrile illness with intravenous drug abuse, positive blood cultures and demonstrable vegetations with tricuspid regurgitation, the most likely diagnosis in this case was of tricuspid valve endocarditis.

CLINICAL DISCUSSION

Endocarditis of the left-sided cardiac valves is more common than that of the right-sided valves. This is because of greater turbulence of blood flow in the left side of the heart and the fact that mitral and aortic valve disease is far more common than tricuspid valve disease. Tricuspid valve endocarditis usually occurs due to intravenous drug abuse. Staphylococcal aureus introduced by contaminated needles from the skin into the venous system, is the most common causative organism (Table 30.1).

Table 30.1: Pathogens implicated in right-sided endocarditis	
• **Typical**	Staphylococcus aureus
• **Atypical**	HACEK* group bacteria
• **Fungal**	Candida, Aspergillus
*HACEK group: Haemophilus, Actinobacillus, Cardiobacterium, Eikenella, Kingella	

Table 30.2: Masses in right atrium
• Right atrial thrombus
• Right atrial myxoma
• Tricuspid vegetation
• Metastatic deposits
• Chiari network remnant
• Eustachian valve of IVC*
* IVC: Inferior Vena Cava

In an immuno-compromised host, HACEK group bacteria and fungal pathogens may be implicated, as in our case. Fungal endocarditis causes large vegetations, which produce a mass in the right atrium. Other causes of a mass in the right atrium are thrombus, myxoma and metastasis (Table 30.2). Tumors that grow along the blood vessels, such as hypernephroma of the kidney and hepato-cellular carcinoma, extend to the right atrium via the inferior vena cava.

The Duke's diagnostic criteria are popularly used for the definite diagnosis of endocarditis. Major criteria are microbiological and echocardiographic criteria. Microbiological evidence is positive blood culture or bacterial serology, of a typical organism consistent with endocarditis. Echocardiographic evidence is endocardial involvement in the form of an oscillating valvular structure or new valvular regurgitation (Table 30.3).

Table 30.3: Diagnostic criteria of infective endocarditis	
Microbiological	• positive blood culture
	• positive bacterial serology
Echocardiographic	• oscillating valvular structure
	• new valvular regurgitation

MANAGEMENT ISSUES

Antimicrobial agents are the mainstay of treatment of infective endocarditis. A bactericidal drug with a low MIC_{90} value against the identified organism is chosen and given intravenously in full doses for an adequate period of time. For Staphylococcal infection, flucloxacillin along with gentamycin is the preferred regimen. For fungal infection, itraconazole or liposomal amphotericin B is chosen. Both these regimens are followed for 4 to 6 weeks. Septic pulmonary emboli which can turn into lung abscess, are treated with antimicrobial drugs and not by anticoagulants.

RECENT ADVANCES

The incidence of Staphylococcal endocarditis has risen due to the widespread use of catheters, venous lines and pacing leads. Methicillin resistant Staph. aureus (MRSA) has emerged as a notorious pathogen. Fungal endocarditis is been recognized in immunocompromised hosts such as HIV-infected patients and organ-transplant recipients on immunosuppressive drugs.

Intracardiac Masses

31

Atrial
Myxoma

CASE PRESENTATION

A 42-year old woman presented to the out-patient department with frequent fainting spells in the preceding two weeks, against a background history of exertional breathlessness. Besides being dyspneic, she had felt fatigued and lethargic over the last 3 months. She had also noticed a low-grade fever and an unintentional weight loss of 4 kg in this period. She gave no history of chills, rigors, night-sweats or nocturnal dyspneic episodes. There was no history of cyanotic spells, squatting attacks or fleeting joint pains during her childhood. She denied smoking tobacco, consuming alcohol or abusing illicit drugs.

On examination, she was mildly pale and dyspneic, but not in any distress. Her heart rate was 96 beats/min. with a BP of 128/84 mm Hg and her temperature was 99.8°F. There were no signs of congestive heart failure. On auscultation, a mid-diastolic rumble was heard at the mitral area, preceded by a high-pitched third heart sound. The intensity and character of the murmur changed with the patient's position. There were no crepitations over the lung fields.

CLINICAL DISCUSSION

A history of dyspnea, constitutional symptoms and febrile illness with a cardiac murmur, raises several diagnostic possibilities. These are:
- Rheumatic fever
- Infective endocarditis
- Connective tissue disorder
- Occult malignant disease
- Atrial myxoma.

The most likely reason for a mid-diastolic murmur in the mitral area is rheumatic mitral stenosis. The murmur is preceded by an opening snap, if the leaflets are pliable. The murmur is best audible with the patient in the left lateral position but does not change its character. ECG and X-ray chest of this patient were unremarkable. ECHO revealed a round mobile mass in the left atrium, arising from the fossa ovalis of the inter-atrial septum and prolapsing into the mitral valve orifice (Fig. 31.1). The mass was lobulated in outline and variegated

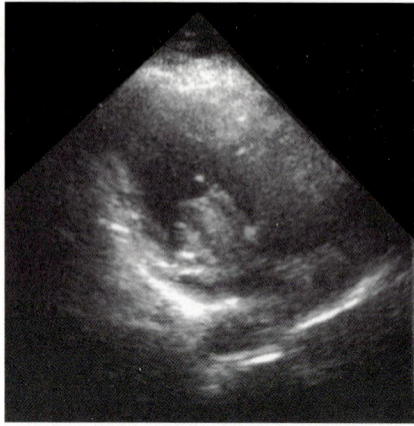

Figure 31.1: ECHO showing left atrial myxoma
prolapsing into the mitral orifice

in echogenicity. The left atrium was mildly dilated but the mitral valve leaflets were normal in structure and excursion. This appearance was highly suggestive of an atrial myxoma.

An atrial thrombus closely resembles a myxoma with certain subtle differences. The thrombus arises from the posterior atrial wall, not the septum and it is never pedunculated. A myxoma is usually pedunculated and rarely sessile. Myxoma generally prolapses into the mitral valve orifice in diastole (Fig. 31.2), unless it is too large in size or sessile. Thrombus is fairly rounded in outline and uniform in echogenicty, while a myxoma is often lobulated and variegated in appearance due to areas of hemorrhage, cystic necrosis and calcification. Moreover, a left atrial thrombus is often associated with structural abnormality of the mitral valve. The differences between an atrial myxoma and an atrial thrombus are given in Table 31.1. Besides an atrial myxoma and an atrial thrombus, other structures that may be rarely seen in the left atrium are supravalvular ring (cor triatriatum), dilated coronary sinus, anomalous pulmonary veins, and large mitral leaflet vegetations.

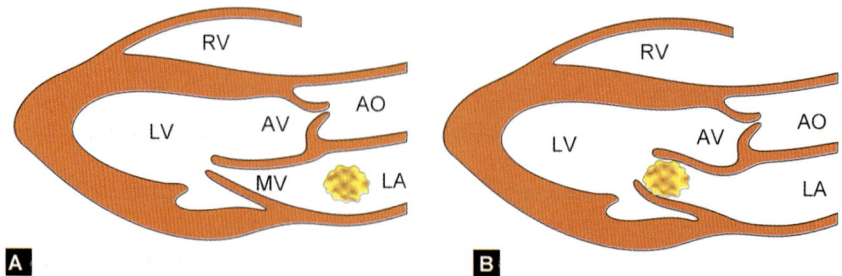

Figure 31.2: Figure showing left atrial myxoma (A), prolapsing into the mitral orifice (B)
RV: Right ventricle; LV: Left ventricle; AV: Aortic valve; MV: Mitral valve;
AO: Aorta; LA: Left atrium

Table 31.1: Differences between atrial myxoma and atrial thrombus		
	Atrial myxoma	**Atrial thrombus**
Site	Atrial septum	Posterior wall
Attachment	Pedunculated	Free
Shape	Lobulated	Rounded
Echogenicity	Echolucent	Echogenic
Prolapse in MV	Often	Rare
Mitral valve	Normal	Diseased

In retrospect, the mid-diastolic murmur in our case was not due to mitral stenosis but caused by the atrial myxoma obstructing the mitral valve (ball-valve effect). Also, the third heart sound preceding the murmur was not the opening snap of the valve but the 'tumour-plop' of the myxoma. On M-mode scan of the mitral valve, there is an early echo-free zone, before the myxoma obstructs the valve. This echo-free zone is not seen in case of mitral stenosis.

In general, cardiac tumours are rare. Secondary metastases are far more common than primary neoplasms of the heart. Metastasis from lung and breast are the commonest due to their overall prevalence and direct extension to the heart (Table 31.2). Majority (75%) of primary cardiac tumours are benign of which nearly half (50%) are myxomas. Other benign tumours are rhabdomyoma and fibroelastoma. Majority of the malignant tumours are the sarcomas such as a rhabdomyosarcoma and fibrosarcoma.

Table 31.2: Various types of cardiac tumours		
Primary (rare)	**Benign** (common)	Myxoma
		Rhabdomyoma
		Fibroelastoma
	Malignant (rare)	Angiosarcoma
		Fibrosarcoma
		Rhabdomyosarcoma
Secondary (common)	**Metastasis**	Lung, breast
		Stomach, ovary
		Lymphoma

A myxoma is a friable and gelatinous tumour of connective tissue origin, related to germ-line mutation. It is more common (75%) in women than men and is generally diagnosed in the fourth or fifth decade of life. It occurs 3 times more often in the left atrium than in the right atrium. Although usually single and 2 to 8 cm in size, myxomas may also be multiple, familial and part of a clinical syndrome with neurofibromas, naevi and lentigines.

NAME syndrome: **N**aevi, **A**trial myxoma, **M**yxoid neurofibroma, **E**philides

LAMB syndrome: **L**entigines, **A**trial **M**yxoma, **B**lue naevi

Myxomas may present with any or all of the triad of symptoms which are constitutional, obstructive and embolic in nature. Systemic symptoms may be vague and include low grade fever, lethargy, arthralgias and weight loss. Obstructive symptoms are due to mitral inflow occlusion and resemble the symptoms of mitral stenosis such as pulmonary congestion, hemoptysis and syncope. Finally, fragments of myxoma tissue may embolize to remote vascular locations.

PERTINENT INVESTIGATIONS

Transesophageal echocardiography (TEE) may provide vital additional information, over and above that obtained from the transthoracic approach. This pertains to the size, site, attachment of the myxoma and its valvular involvement. This information serves as a guide for surgical resection. Advanced imaging techniques such as computed tomography (CT) and magnetic resonance imaging (MRI), provide further useful anatomical information.

MANAGEMENT ISSUES

Surgical resection of the myxoma is the only definitive form of treatment and most myxomas are amenable to surgery. Complete full thickness resection is preferable, in order to prevent recurrence. Myxomas are removed even if they do not cause any symptoms, in order to avoid embolic events. The atrial septum to which the myxoma is often attached, is reconstructed using a pericardial patch. Long-term surveillance by annual follow-up ECHO is recommended to detect recurrence.

RECENT ADVANCES

Newer sophisticated imaging techniques such as computed tomography (CT) and magnetic resonance imaging (MRI) can improve upon the anatomical information about myxomas provided by echocardiography (ECHO). More recently, contrast ECHO has been used to differentiate myxomas from thrombi on the basis of their vascularity. Intravenous injection of microbubbles will perfuse the tumour but not the thrombus.

32

Atrial Thrombus

CASE PRESENTATION

A 32-year old married woman, a domestic servant by profession, came to a general hospital with sudden weakness of the right hand and inability to walk, since the last 10 hours. There was no history of recent febrile illness, trauma to the head or purulent discharge from the ear. However, she always felt tired and short of breath and she had curtailed her working hours for the past 1 year. She also experienced episodic palpitations and dizzy spells, ever since the birth of her second child, 3 years back. She recollected being extremely breathless in the last trimester of her pregnancy and her obstetrician strictly advising her not to bear any more children. The patient also distinctly remembered having been incapacitated by severe joint pains for over a month, when she was 15 years of age.

On examination, she was anxious and tachypneic. Her tongue and palms were pale but there was no cyanosis or icterus. The pulse was irregular, low in volume at a rate of about 90 beats/min. while the heart rate was around 110 beats/min. The BP was 104/72 mm Hg in the right arm and all peripheral pulses were palpable. The JVP was raised and there was mild pitting edema over the ankles. The apex beat was normal in character and a left parasternal heave was felt. The S_1 was variable in intensity and the P_2 was loudly audible. A low-pitched mid-diastolic rumble was heard over the cardiac apex, which did not accentuate in pre-systole. The lung fields were clear on auscultation. On neurological examination, power in the right hand and at the elbow was grade 3 while power in the right knee was grade 4. Sensations were preserved and the deep tendon reflexes were diminished on the right side. The was also a right supranuclear facial nerve palsy and slight slurring of speech.

CLINICAL DISCUSSION

From the history and physical examination, this woman had rheumatic heart disease with mitral stenosis and atrial fibrillation. In all likelihood, she had an embolic stroke due to a dislodged fragment of a left atrial thrombus, which occluded the left middle cerebral artery and caused hemiparesis. An irregular pulse, with a pulse rate deficit compared to the heart rate, are signs of atrial fibrillation. The S_1 is variable in intensity, because of a beat-to-beat variation of the diastolic filling period. In the presence of atrial fibrillation, the mid-diastolic murmur does not undergo presystolic accentuation, because the atrial contribution to ventricular filling is absent.

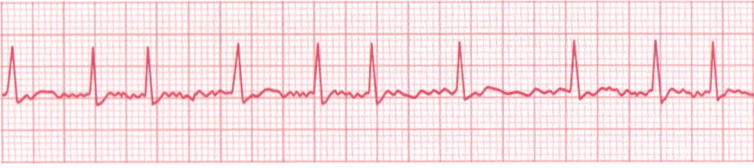

Figure 32.1: ECG showing atrial fibrillation with fast ventricular response

As expected, the ECG showed atrial fibrillation with a fast ventricular response (Fig. 32.1). Additionally, there was evidence of right ventricular hypertrophy and right-ward deviation of the QRS vector. X-ray chest findings were cardiomegaly, straightening of the left heart border with a prominent atrial appendage as well as signs of interstitial pulmonary edema. On ECHO, the left ventricle was normal but the left atrium and right ventricle were dilated. The mitral valve leaflets were thickened and showed limited excursion with diastolic doming (Fig. 32.2). The aortic valve was structurally normal. No mass or thrombus was demonstrated in any cardiac chamber. The pulmonary artery pressure, as estimated from the tricuspid regurgitant jet, was elevated.

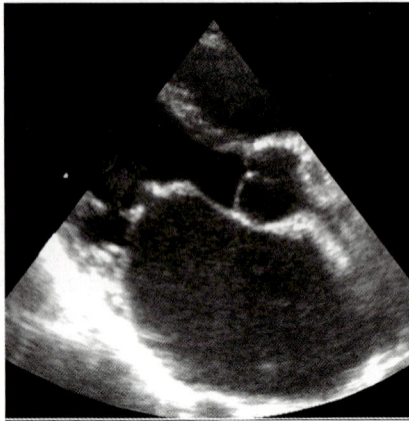

Figure 32.2: ECHO showing thickened mitral leaflets, diastolic doming and dilated left atrium

Enlargement of the left atrial appendage is typical of mitral valve disease, be it stenosis or regurgitation, especially when due to rheumatic heart disease. Probably acute rheumatic carditis damages the left atrial wall and its appendage, causing them to bulge when the atrial filling pressure rises. Enlargement of the left atrial appendage causes straightening of the left heart border on chest X-ray (Fig. 32.3). The "4-bump heart" is formed above downward by the aortic knuckle, pulmonary artery, left atrial appendage and the left ventricular lateral wall.

The risk of thromboembolism in mitral stenosis is very high, particularly if atrial fibrillation is present and more so if it is intermittent. Mitral stenosis can be safely assumed to be the cause of cerebral infarction, even if a left atrial thrombus is not demonstrable. A thrombus that is too small for detection, thrombus in the atrial appendage or one that has already embolised, may be missed on

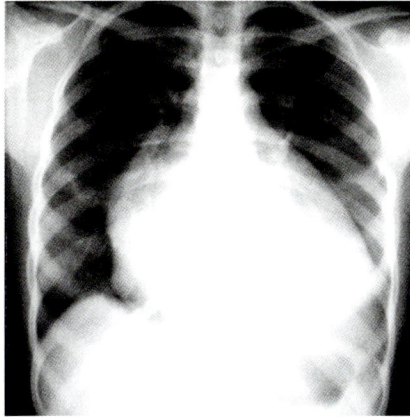

Figure 32.3: X-RAY showing cardiomegaly with
straightening of left heart border

transthoracic echo. Transesophageal echocardiography (TEE) vastly improves
the detection of a thrombus in the left atrial cavity or its appendage. Occasionally,
an ECHO may show a very large atrial thrombus, which is potentially fatal if it
suddenly obstructs the mitral valve. Such a 'ball-valve' thrombus is an indication
for urgent surgical intervention.

A left atrial thrombus sometimes needs to be differentiated from a left atrial
myxoma, since both can cause distal embolism. Thrombus usually arises from the
posterior atrial wall or floats freely, while myxoma is usually pedunculated and is
attached to the inter-atrial septum. Thrombus is rounded in shape and uniform
in echogenicity, while myxoma is often lobulated with variable echogenicity due
to areas of hemorrhage, necrosis or calcification. Finally, thrombus uncommonly
prolapses into the diseased mitral valve while myxoma commonly prolapses
into the normal mitral valve. The differences between atrial thrombus and atrial
myxoma are given in Table 32.1.

Besides an atrial thrombus and an atrial myxoma, other structures that may be
sometimes seen in the left atrium are supravalvular ring (cor triatriatum), dilated
coronary sinus, anomalous pulmonary veins, large mitral leaflet vegetation and
reverberation artefacts from a calcified mitral annulus.

Table 32.1: Differences between atrial thrombus and atrial myxoma		
	Atrial thrombus	**Atrial myxoma**
Site	Posterior wall	Atrial septum
Attachment	Free	Pedunculated
Shape	Rounded	Lobulated
Echogenicity	Echogenic	Echolucent
Prolapse in MV	Rare	Often
Mitral valve	Diseased	Normal

MANAGEMENT ISSUES

In a patient of mitral stenosis and atrial fibrillation with a thrombo-embolic stroke, the first priority is anticoagulation. Low molecular-weight heparin(LMWH) such as enoxaparin is preferred because of predictable pharmacokinetics, without the need of prothrombin time (PT) and aPTT monitoring. An oral anticoagulant like warfarin is initiated almost simultaneously, since it requires 3 to 5 days to produce optimal anticoagulation. Oral anticoagulation is required on a long-term basis in a patient of mitral stenosis with history of thromboembolism.

Other cardiovascular drugs are used to reduce the symptomatology of mitral stenosis. Diuretics reduce pulmonary congestion, especially in those with concomitant mitral regurgitation. Digoxin, beta-blockers and verapamil control the ventricular response in atrial fibrillation and improve left ventricular diastolic filling. Percutanenous balloon mitral valvuloplasty (BMV) in not advocated in patients with a demonstrable left atrial thrombus. Mitral valve replacement is required for critical stenosis (mitral valve area < 1 cm^2).

CASE
33

Ventricular Thrombus

A 67-year old gentleman was brought to the cardiology department by his son for a follow-up visit, 1 week after discharge from the hospital. The patient had sustained an anterior wall myocardial infarction 2 weeks ago, for which he received thrombolytic therapy. However, the streptokinase infusion was stopped at the half-way stage, because the patient developed hypotension. Thereafter, his course in the hospital was by-and-large uneventful, barring a extrasystolic ventricular bigeminy lasting 36 hours, which was treated with lignocaine infusion. Upon returning home, he did not experience any angina, dyspnea, palpitation or syncope. Medications prescribed to him were aspirin 150 mg, clopidogrel 75 mg, ramipril 5 mg, atorvastatin 20 mg and metoprolol 50 mg.

On examination, the patient was alert, comfortable and not tachypneic. The pulse was fair in volume, at a rate of 92 beats/min. and few ectopic beats were noticed. The BP was 110/66 mm Hg in the right arm. All peripheral pulses were well palpable. The JVP was not raised and there was no hepatomegaly or ankle edema. On precordial examination, the apex beat was diffuse in nature and displaced towards the left axilla. The S_1 and S_2 heart sounds were normal but a soft S_3 was audible in diastole. There was no murmur or pericardial rub audible. Few inspiratory crackles were heard over the lower lung fields posteriorly.

ECG showed sinus rhythm at a rate of 92 beats/min. and an occasional unifocal ventricular premature beat was seen. No couplet or bigeminal rhythm was noticed. There was complete attenuation of the R waves with deep Q waves in the precordial leads V_1 to V_4. Small q waves were also seen in leads V_5 and V_6 (Fig. 33.1). There was coving of the S-T segment with inversion of the T wave in all the precordial leads. The Q-T interval was normal.

ECHO showed a dilated left ventricle with depressed systolic function (ejection fraction 35%). The mid and distal segments of the interventricular septum, the left ventricular apex and the distal segment of the lateral wall were hypokinetic but no dyskinetic area was identified. A well-defined rounded mass was seen arising from the ventricular apex and protruding into the left ventricular cavity (Fig. 33.2). The echogenicity of the mass was variable and it did not move in synchrony with the ventricle. The posterior mitral leaflet failed to reach the plane of the mitral annulus and the leaflet coaptation point was distally located in the ventricle. The aortic valve leaflets were mildly thickened but had normal excursion without systolic doming. No pericardial effusion was noted.

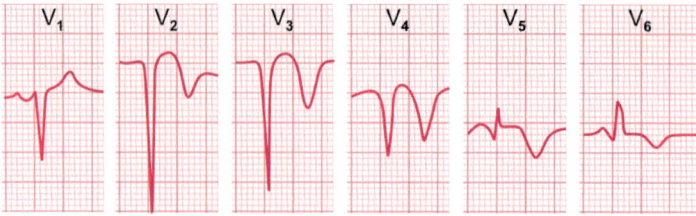

Figure 33.1: ECG showing R wave attenuation, deep Q waves with S-T segment coving and T wave inversion

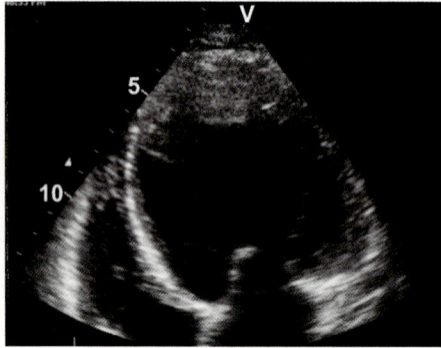

Figure 33.2: ECHO showing a dilated, hypokinetic left ventricle with a mural thrombus arising from the apex

CLINICAL DISCUSSION

From the history and physical examination as well as from the ECG and ECHO findings, this elderly gentleman had sustained a recent extensive anterior wall myocardial infarction. He had now developed left ventricular systolic dysfunction and a ventricular thrombus. Two weeks after acute myocardial infarction (MI) usual complications include post-MI angina, malignant ventricular arrhythmias and left ventricular failure. Sometimes, a ventricular thrombus may form on an infarcted and scarred myocardial segment or within a left ventricular aneurysm. This patient did not demonstrate any dyskinetic myocardial segment and there was no outward bulge of the left ventricular cavity. A fragment of the ventricular thrombus may break away and travel through the systemic circulation to cause embolization in any distal vascular bed.

A dilated left ventricle with reduced systolic wall motion and stagnated blood flow, is an ideal setting for ventricular thrombus formation. A ventricular thrombus may form on a dyskinetic, infarcted and scarred myocardial segment or within a left ventricular aneurysm. Idiopathic dilated cardiomyopathy is another important reason for ventricular thrombus formation.

A pedunculated ventricular thrombus appears as a well-defined, rounded, mobile stalked mass, that protrudes into the ventricular cavity. The mobility of the thrombus is not synchronous with the left ventricular free wall motion. It is more likely to embolize if the echodensity is variable due to areas of necrosis. A mural ventricular thrombus is a flat, laminated mass, contiguous with the ventricular wall with which it moves synchronously. It is more echogenic than the adjacent myocardium and less likely to embolize than a pedunculated thrombus. Thrombus always has a clear identifiable edge while an artefact caused by stagnated blood has a hazy appearance. On color flow mapping, the flow stops abruptly at the edge of a thrombus but not at the edge of an artefact.

Left ventricular thrombus is a masquerader of several other mass lesions. Causes of a mass in the left ventricle are rhabdomyoma, false tendon and prominent papillary muscle. Mural thrombus can be distinguished from localized myocardial thickening by the fact that myocardium thickens during systole while a thrombus does not. Thrombus can be differentiated from a cardiac tumor by the fact that adjacent wall motion is almost always abnormal in case of thrombus and often normal in case of tumor.

MANAGEMENT ISSUES

Presence of a ventricular thrombus is an established indication for oral anticoagulant therapy. Other clear indications for anticoagulation are mechanical prosthetic heart valve, left atrial thrombus with mitral stenosis and ventricular aneurysm. When an oral anticoagulant like warfarin is initiated, it takes 3 to 5 days for the onset of full therapeutic effect. In this interim period, heparin therapy may be given. Unfractionated heparin requires monitoring but it is cost effective. Low molecular weight heparin (LMWH) is more expensive, but it does not require prothrombin time (PT) or aPTT monitoring.

It is now widely recommended that every myocardial infarction patient must receive aspirin, a statin, an ACE-inhibitor and a beta-blocker. Our patient had already been prescribed all these drugs. A diuretic can be added to reduce cardiac work-load, if pulmonary congestive symptoms develop. An aldosterone antagonist such as spironolactone or eplerenone can also be used. These drugs, besides reducing cardiac work-load, improve ventricular remodelling and lower cardiovascular mortality.

Typical ECG Abnormalities

Left Ventricular Hypertrophy

CASE PRESENTATION

A 56-year old obese gentleman visited his physician with the complaints of frequent headaches and spells of dizziness. He also found it difficult to carry out routine tasks and felt fatigued and breathless even on mild physical exertion. The patient was diagnosed to have systemic hypertension about 30 years back. At that time, he was extensively investigated for secondary hypertension, but no renal or endocrine disorder was detected. He was prescribed antihypertensive medications, but did not take them regularly and was not on periodic medical follow-up. The patient had always been overweight even at a young age and was diagnosed to have diabetes mellitus about 10 years back. He had not got his lipid profile checked recently. The man was sedentary and did not follow any particular diet plan. He smoked 8 to 10 cigarettes per day and consumed 2 to 3 large pegs of whiskey, on most days of the week.

On examination, the patient was grossly overweight, with a body mass index (BMI) of 34 kg/m². He was tachypneic and afebrile. The pulse was regular, good in volume and the heart rate was 84 beats/min. All peripheral pulses were palpable and there was no carotid bruit or brachio-femoral delay. The BP was 164/106 mm Hg over the right arm in the sitting position. The JVP was not raised but mild edema was present over the ankles. The cardiac apex beat was sustained and heaving in nature and systolic pulsations were observed in the suprasternal notch. The S₁ was normal but the A₂ sound was accentuated; a S₄ sound was heard in presystole. A soft systolic murmur was audible over the upper left parasternal area. Few basilar rales were audible over the lung fields. An ECG was obtained (Fig. 34.1).

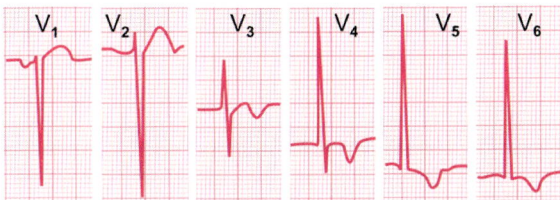

Figure 34.1: ECG showing tall R waves in left chest leads
with deep S waves in right chest leads

ECG INTERPRETATION

The ECG showed tall R waves exceeding 25 mm in the left precordial leads and deep S waves in the right precordial leads. There also was S-T segment depression and T-wave inversion in the lateral leads. These findings are consistent with the diagnosis of left ventricular hypertrophy. The tall R waves in the lateral precordial leads, reflect the increased electrical forces generated by the thickened left ventricular myocardium. S-T segment depression and T wave inversion in these leads indicate left ventricular strain. Additional findings can include notched bifid P waves (P. mitrale) due to left atrial enlargement and left axis deviation of the QRS vector.

Voltage criteria are often employed for the electrical diagnosis of left ventricular hypertrophy (Table 34.1). The Sokolow and Lyon criteria of S in V_1 plus R in V_5 or V_6 greater than 35 mm is popularly used. Another criteria used is of Framingham wherein, R in V_5 or V_6 >25 mm or R in aVL >11 mm is taken as criteria for left ventricular hypertrophy. The left ventricular (LV) strain pattern of S-T segment depression and T-wave inversion is observed in LV pressure overload. In case of LV volume overload, the S-T segment is isoelectric and the T wave is upright and tall.

Table 34.1: Voltage criteria for left ventricular hypertrophy
• **Sokolow and Lyon Criteria** S. in V_1 + R in V_5 or V_6 >35 mm
• **Framingham Criteria** R in V_5 or V_6 >25 mm; R in aVL >11 mm

CLINICAL DISCUSSION

Causes of left ventricular hypertrophy are classified into those of systolic overload and the causes of diastolic overload. Systolic overload is due to systemic hypertension, aortic stenosis, coarctation of aorta and hypertrophic cardiomyopathy. Causes of diastolic overload are mitral and aortic valve regurgitation and an intracardiac left-to-right shunt such as ventricular septal defect or patent ductus arteriosus (Table 34.2).

Echocardiography is 5 to 10 times more sensitive than an ECG, in detecting left ventricular hypertrophy (LVH). Presence of LVH is the most common ECHO abnormality in a hypertensive patient. Conversely, systemic hypertension is the most common cause of LVH. Besides detecting LVH, ECHO is used to evaluate left ventricular systolic and diastolic function and for the diagnosis of associated coronary artery disease. Other abnormalities seen on ECHO are mitral and aortic valve degeneration, dilatation of the aortic root and rarely aortic coarctation (Table 34.3). ECHO typically shows thickening of the interventricular septum (IVS) and LV posterior wall (LVPW) greater than 11 mm with virtual obliteration of the left ventricular cavity during systole (Fig. 34.2). Left ventricular hypertrophy is an

Table 34.2: Causes of left ventricular hypertrophy

Systolic overload
- Aortic valve stenosis
- Systemic hypertension
- Coarctation of the aorta
- Hypertrophic cardiomyopathy

Diastolic overload
- Mitral regurgitation
- Aortic incompetence
- Ventricular septal defect
- Patent ductus arteriosus.

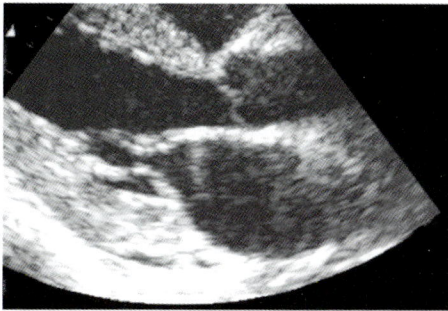

Figure 34.2: ECHO showing thick septum and posterior wall with obliteration of left ventricular cavity

independent predictor of cardiovascular morbidity and mortality, as a risk factor for myocardial infarction, stroke, heart failure and sudden arrhythmic death. Serial echoes are performed annually to monitor the progress of hypertensive heart disease, particularly to assess the regression of LVH with antihypertensive drug therapy.

Table 34.3: ECHO findings in systemic hypertension

- Left ventricular hypertrophy (LVH)
- Diastolic and systolic LV dysfunction
- Regional wall motion abnormality
- Mitral and aortic valve calcification
- Dilatation of aortic root
- Coarctation of aorta.

MANAGEMENT ISSUES

Current practice guidelines recommend that all hypertensive patients with left ventricular hypertrophy, target organ damage and associated cardiovascular risk factors particularly diabetes, should be offered antihypertensive drug treatment. The choice of first-line therapy has been the subject of debate, as well as the study design of several clinical trials. It is being believed that newer agents like calcium channel blockers (e.g. amlodipine) or an ACE inhibitor (e.g. ramipril) are more effective for regression of hypertrophy than older agents like diuretics (e.g. thiazide) or beta blockers (e.g. atenolol). Moreover, newer agents are less likely to increase the risk of diabetes than the older agents. The increased risk of diabetes with older drugs is particularly relevant in patients of South Asian origin, who are already at higher risk of developing diabetes and the metabolic syndrome.

Left Bundle Branch Block

CASE PRESENTATION

A 63-year old man was brought to the emergency room past midnight, with the complaint of shortness of breath and difficulty in lying flat on the bed. The patient had sustained an anterior wall myocardial infarction 5 months back and ever since, he had complained of easy fatiguability and dyspnea on exertion. For the past 1 week, he required 2 or 3 pillows in bed to catch sleep and yet woke up often because of air-hunger. There was no recent history of chest pain, palpitation or syncope. His current daily medication was ramipril 5 mg, torsemide 20 mg, metoprolol 25 mm, aspirin 150 mg, clopidogrel 75 mg and atorvastatin 10 mg.

On examination, the patient was obviously tachypneic and looked anxious. He was pale and diaphoretic. The extremities were cold but there was no cyanosis. The JVP was not raised and there was no pitting edema around the ankles. The pulse was fast and low in volume with variable volume in successive beats. The BP was 104/74 mm Hg over the right arm in the supine position. The cardiac apex beat was diffuse and displaced towards the left axilla. The S_1 was normal and the A_2 was loud. There was paradoxical splitting of S_2, that shortened during the phase of inspiration. A S_3 was also appreciated in early diastole. A pansystolic murmur was audible over the cardiac apex, that radiated towards the axilla. Auscultation over the lung fields revealed bilateral crepts over the bases posteriorly. An ECG was obtained (Fig. 35.1).

ECG INTERPRETATION

The ECG showed broad ventricular complexes, that measured 0.14 sec. in width. In leads L_1 and V_6, each ventricular complex had two peaks, producing a M-shaped RsR' pattern. The broad complex was followed by S-T segment depression and T-wave inversion. These findings are consistent with the diagnosis of left bundle branch block. Bundle branch block denotes delayed or interrupted conduction down the right or left branch of the bundle of His (Fig. 35.2). It leads to widening of the ventricular complex, due to delayed depolarization of the ventricle whose bundle branch is blocked. The QRS complexes of both the ventricles are "out of sync" with each other and produce two R waves in sequential order. Incomplete bundle branch block (BBB) results in QRS width of 0.11 to 0.12 sec while in complete BBB, the QRS width exceeds 0.12 sec. The S-T segment depression and

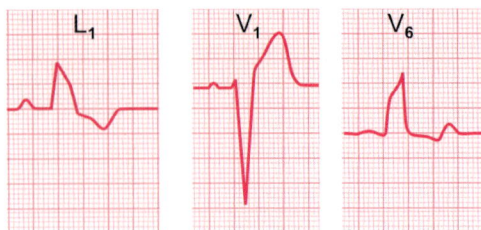

Figure 35.1: ECG showing wide QRS complexes due to left bundle branch block

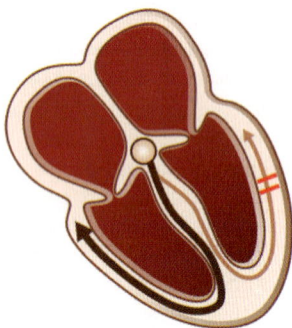

Figure 35.2: Diagram to represent left bundle branch block (LBBB)

T-wave inversion are repolarization abnormalities, secondary to the abnormal pattern of ventricular depolarization.

In left bundle branch block (LBBB), the M-shaped RsR' pattern is observed in lead V_6. The notched R wave represents abnormal sequence of septal and left ventricular free wall depolarization. There is total distortion of the normal QRS complex. In right bundle branch block (RBBB), the M-shaped rsR pattern is observed in lead V_1. The septal (denoted by r) and free wall (denoted by S) depolarization through the left bundle branch are normal. Right ventricular depolarization (denoted by R') is delayed. Therefore RBBB does not distort the normal QRS complex, but only adds a terminal R' deflection.

Block in the conduction of impulses down one of the two fascicles of the left bundle branch constitutes a hemiblock (Fig. 35.3). Left anterior hemiblock (LAHB) is far more common than left posterior hemiblock (LPHB). Anterior hemiblock is more common because the anterior fascicle is compact, has a single blood-supply and lies close to the disease prone aortic valve. On the other hand, the posterior fascicle is fan-like, has a dual blood-supply and is far less likely to be involved in septal pathology. Hemiblock (LAHB) causes an abnormal pattern of left ventricular activation, resulting in left axis deviation of the QRS vector (Fig. 35.4).

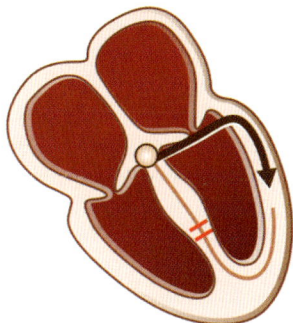

Figure 35.3: Diagram to represent left anterior hemiblock (LAHB)

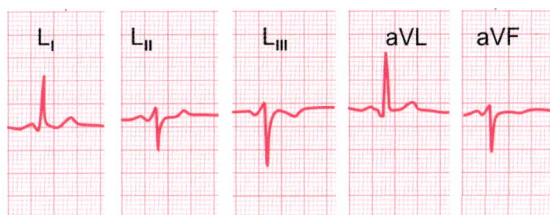

Figure 35.4: ECG showing left axis deviation due to left anterior hemiblock

CLINICAL DISCUSSION

Left bundle branch block (LBBB) often indicates the presence of organic heart disease. A variety of cardiac conditions can cause LBBB including myocardial infarction, systemic hypertension, aortic valve disease, cardiomyopathy and fibrocalcerous degeneration (Table 35.1). On the other hand, right bundle branch block (RBBB) is sometimes observed in normal individuals. Typical causes of RBBB are atrial septal defect, acute pulmonary embolism and chronic obstructive pulmonary disease.

RBBB does not distort the QRS complex, but only adds a terminal deflection due to delayed right ventricular depolarization. Therefore, changes of myocardial infarction such as appearance of Q waves and loss of R wave height, can be readily diagnosed in the presence of RBBB. However, it is difficult to diagnose myocardial infarction in the presence of LBBB, since the QRS complex is completely distorted.

Table 35.1: Causes of left bundle branch block
• Myocardial infarction
• Aortic valve stenosis
• Systemic hypertension
• Dilated cardiomyopathy
• Fibrocalcerous degeneration.

> **Table 35.2: Criteria for diagnosing MI in presence of LBBB**
>
> - Presence of q wave in L_1, V_5 and V_6
> - Terminal S wave in leads V_5 and V_6
> - S-T segment drift greater than 5mm
> - Upright T wave concordant with QRS

The criteria for the diagnosis of myocardial infarction in the presence of LBBB are given in Table 35.2.

In left bundle branch block (LBBB), there is paradoxical splitting of the second heart sound (S_2). The A_2 component of S_2 is delayed due to late depolarization of the left ventricle and follows the P_2. During inspiration, when P_2 gets delayed due to increased venous return, the splitting of S_2 becomes narrow instead of physiological widening. Besides LBBB, another cause of paradoxical splitting of S_2 is aortic valve stenosis in which left ventricular ejection time is prolonged. Other reasons for paradoxical splitting of A_2 are pre-excitation of the right ventricle through an accessory bypass tract or premature activation of the right ventricle by an external pacemaker. LBBB causes a jerky motion of the interventricular septum on echocardiography. This should not be diagnosed as septal infarction, unless the septum fails to thicken during systole.

MANAGEMENT ISSUES

There is no specific treatment of left bundle branch block. The underlying heart disease is to be managed on its own merit. There is a word of caution regarding the use of drugs which block the A-V node such as verapamil, diltiazem and beta blockers. They may cause complete heart block, particularly if the block is bifascicular or trifascicular to begin with. Bifasicular block includes right bundle branch block and left anterior hemiblock. Trifasicular block is bifasicular block with a prolonged P-R interval.

36

Features of Hypokalemia

CASE PRESENTATION

A 48-year old man sought consultation from a physician for pain and weakness in both arms, since the last 3 days. There was no history of chest pain, breathlessness, palpitation or sweating. The heaviness in the arms was aggravated by lifting a light weight, but not by movement at the neck. The patient also complained of fatigue and pain over his calf muscles while walking. He had systemic hypertension for several years for which he was presently prescribed losartan 50 mg and hydrochlorthiazide 25 mg. The patient also suffered from bronchial asthma, for which he used an inhaler containing a combination of salmeterol and fluticasone. Recently, he had a gastro-intestinal infection with profuse vomiting and diarrhea that lasted 2 days. Besides age and hypertension, other cardiovascular risk factors in the patient were prediabetes and a modestly elevated serum cholesterol.

On examination, the patient was coherent, comfortable and in no distress. There was no anemia, cyanosis, icterus or ankle edema. The JVP was not raised, thyroid gland was normal and there were no palpable lymph-nodes. The pulse rate was 72 beats/min with a BP of 130/80 mm Hg. The precordium was unremarkable and the apex beat was normally located. The S_1 and S_2 were normal and no gallop sound was heard. No murmur or pericardial friction rub was audible. The breath sounds were normal without rhonchi or crepts. An ECG was obtained (Fig. 36.1) following which he was asked to immediately see a cardiologist. His blood biochemistry was Glucose 128 mg/dl, Urea 38 mg/dl, Creatinine 1.2 mg/dl, LDL cholesterol 147 mg/dl, Sodium 131 m Eq/L and Potassium 2.9 m Eq/L.

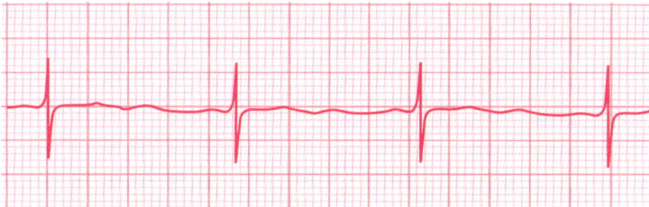

Figure 36.1: ECG showing flat T waves with prominent U waves

ECG INTERPRETATION

The ECG showed normal sinus rhythm. The P wave and QRS complex were normal in morphology. There were no significant Q waves and the S-T segment was isoelectric. The T wave was reduced in amplitude, while the U wave was prominent. The Q-T interval seemed to be prolonged. These findings are consistent with the diagnosis of hypokalemia. Hypokalemia is an important cause of T wave change. The T wave is either reduced in amplitude, flattened or inverted. This is associated with prominence of the U wave that follows the T wave. The low T wave followed by a prominent U wave produces a 'camel-hump' effect.

In hypokalemia, the T wave is flattened and the prominent U wave may be mistaken for the T wave. This may falsely suggest prolongation of the Q-T interval, whereas it is actually the Q-U interval. Hypokalemia therefore causes pseudo-prolongation of the Q-T interval, at the expense of T wave. The U wave that is exaggerated and approximates the size of the T wave is considered to be a prominent U wave. Other causes of prominent U wave are cardiovascular drugs e.g. digitalis, quinidine and psychotropic agents e.g. phenothiazines, tricyclic antidepressants.

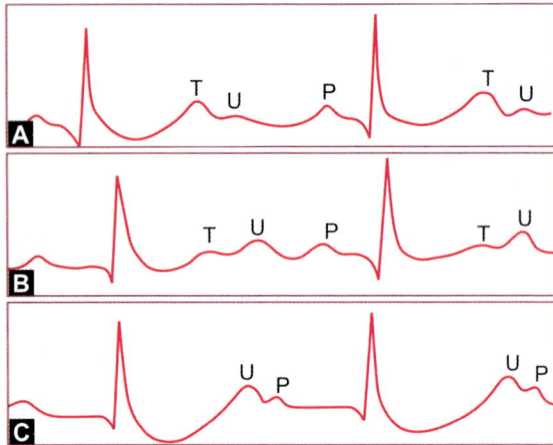

Figure 36.2: ECG features of progressively increasing hypokalemia

The ECG features of hypokalemia depend upon its severity (Fig. 36.2). In mild hypokalemia, only the T wave amplitude is reduced. In moderate hypokalemia, the U wave becomes more prominent than the T wave. In severe hypokalemia, there is sagging of the S-T segment and only the U wave is visible (Table 36.1).

Table 36.1: ECG features of progressive hypokalemia
• Reduced amplitude of the T wave
• Flat T wave with prominent U wave
• S-T segment sagging; only U wave.

CLINICAL DISCUSSION

The ECG is sometimes helpful in the diagnosis of an electrolyte abnormality, even before the blood biochemistry results from the laboratory are available. Variation in the blood levels of potassium and calcium are mainly responsible for these ECG changes. Hypokalemia causes pseudo-prolongation of the Q-T interval, at the expense of the T wave. Hypocalcemia causes true prolongation of the Q-T interval, with true lengthening of the S-T segment.

Table 36.2: Causes of hypokalemia
• **Body fluid loss** Diuresis Vomiting Diarrhea
• **Redistribution** Metabolic alkalosis
• **Drug-induced** Beta-agonist Insulin therapy
• **Hyperaldosteronism** Cushing's disease Conn's syndrome
• **Genetic causes** Hypokalemic periodic paralysis Renal tubular acidosis Type 2

There are several causes of hypokalemia which have been enlisted in Table 36.2. True loss of potassium is due to vomiting, diarrhea, naso-gastric suction and diuretic therapy (see Table 36.2). Redistribution of potassium occurs in metabolic alkalosis (intracellular shift) and with beta-agonist or insulin therapy. Hypokalemia is a feature of cortisol excess due to Cushing's disease or steroid therapy as well as a feature of hyperaldosteronism in Conn's syndrome. Genetic causes of hypokalemia are Type 2 renal tubular acidosis (RTA-2) and hypokalemic periodic paralysis. Typical clinical features of hypokalemia are fatigue and leg cramps. In severe cases, neuromuscular paralysis and cardiac arrhythmias may occur. In cardiac patients on diuretic treatment, hypokalemia aggravates digitalis toxicity and increases the likelihood of serious ventricular arrhythmias.

In our case, the hypokalemia was multi-factorial. Firstly, the patient was prescribed a diuretic for his hypertension. Secondly, he was using an inhaled beta-agonist for asthma, which is known to cause hypokalemia. Finally, he had a recent episode of gastro-enteritis, which might have caused substantial loss of potassium from his body.

Table 36.3: Management of hypokalemia
• **Potassium replacement** Dietary supplements Oral K preparations Intravenous infusion
• **Treatment of the cause** Anti-emetics Anti-diarrheals Diuretic withdrawal

MANAGEMENT ISSUES

Management of hypokalemia includes potassium replacement and correction of the underlying cause (Table 36.3). Potassium can be replaced through dietary supplementation of potassium-rich foods. Oral proprietary supplements of potassium citrate can also be prescribed. If potassium deficiency is severe or if the patient is vomiting, potassium chloride is administered as an intravenous infusion. Generally, potassium deficiency is more severe, if there is true loss of body fluids than if there is only a transcellular shift of potassium.

Features of Hyperkalemia

CASE PRESENTATION

A 64-year old woman was wheeled into the emergency room, with generalized weakness and shortness of breath of one week duration. She also complained of swelling around the eyes and over the feet, loss of appetite and occasional vomiting. The lady was a known case of diabetes mellitus since 25 years and systemic hypertension for the last 12 years. She sustained an anterior wall myocardial infarction four years back, for which she was thrombolysed. At that time, coronary angiography showed triple-vessel disease, but she declined a revascularization procedure. Her serum creatinine value was found to be high and therefore, she was switched over from oral antidiabetic drugs to insulin therapy. The patient also underwent laser photocoagulation for proliferative retinopathy, one year back. She was presently undergoing maintenance hemodialysis, thrice a week.

On examination, the patient was drowsy, disoriented and obviously dyspneic. The complexion was pale and sallow with dry skin that bore marks of pruritus. There was periorbital puffiness and pitting edema over the ankles and lower legs. The neck veins were engorged but there was no cyanosis or icterus. The pulse rate was 92 beats/min. with a BP of 160/94 mm Hg. The precordium was unremarkable and the apex beat was displaced to the left. The S_1 was normal with a loud A_2 and a S_3 sound in early diastole. An ejection murmur was audible along the left sternal border. No pericardial friction rub was audible. There were bilateral basilar rales over the lung fields. An ECG was obtained (Fig. 37.1) following which she was immediately given an injection. Her laboratory reports were Hemoglobin 9.2 g/dL% Urine sugar +1 albumin +2, Glucose 144 mg/dl, Urea 124 mg/dl, Creatinine 5.2 mg/dl, Sodium 129 mEq/L, Potassium 6.8 mEq/L and Calcium 7.4 mg%.

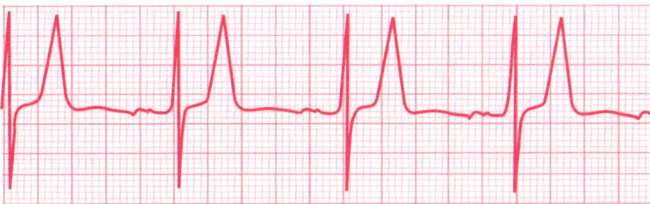

Figure 37.1: ECG showing tall T waves with flat P waves

ECG INTERPRETATION

The ECG showed normal sinus rhythm. The P wave was flattened and the P-R interval was prolonged. There were no significant Q waves and the S-T segment was isoelectric. The T wave was upright, tall and peaked. The Q-T interval was short. These findings are consistent with the diagnosis of hyperkalemia. A T-wave that exceeds a voltage of 5 mm in the standard leads and 10 mm in the precordial leads is considered tall. Besides hyperkalemia, causes of tall T wave are myocardial ischemia and the hyperacute phase of myocardial infarction. The T wave of hyperkalemia is tall, peaked symmetrical and has a narrow base, the so called 'tented' T wave. The Q-T interval is short. On the other hand, the T wave of coronary insufficiency is tall but broad-based and the Q-T interval is prolonged.

The normal Q-T interval is 0.39 ± 0.04 sec. and ranges from 0.35 to 0.43 sec. A Q-T interval measuring less than 0.35 sec is considered short. Besides hyperkalemia, causes of short Q-T interval are hypercalcemia and digitalis toxicity. Hyperkalemia shortens the Q-T interval and is associated with tall T waves, wide QRS complexes and diminished P waves. Hypercalcemia also shortens the Q-T interval but there are no changes in the morphology of the QRS deflection. The proximal limb of the T-wave has an abrupt upslope to its peak.

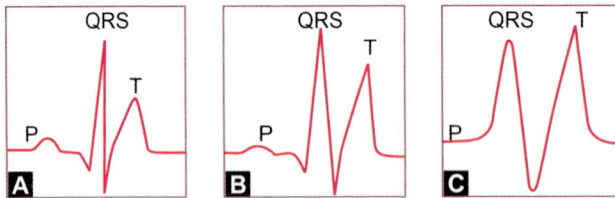

Figure 37.2: ECG features of progressively increasing hyperkalemia

The ECG features of hyperkalemia depend upon its severity (Fig. 37.2). When the serum level exceeds 6.8 mEq/L, tall T waves and short Q-T interval are seen. When it exceeds 8.4 mEq/L, additionally the P wave gets flattened and the P-R interval gets prolonged. At a serum level which is in excess of 9.1 mEq/L, the QRS complex also becomes wide and ventricular arrhythmias occur (Table 37.1).

Table 37.1: ECG features of progressive hyperkalemia		
A.	Serum K>6.8 mEq/L	tall T waves; short Q-T interval
B.	Serum K>8.4 mEq/L	(A) plus flat P waves; prolonged P-R interval
C.	Serum K>9.1 mEq/L	(B) plus wide QRS complex; A-V block and arrhythmias

CLINICAL DISCUSSION

The electrocardiogram often shows changes due to an electrolyte abnormality. These changes are observed even before the biochemical reports from the laboratory are available. Variation in the blood levels of potassium and calcium are chiefly responsible for these ECG changes. Abnormal levels of calcium and magnesium produce similar changes. Hypercalcemia shortens the Q-T interval while hypocalcemia prolongs it.

Table 37.2: Causes of hyperkalemia
• **Potassium gain**   Hemolysis, tumour lysis   Rhabdomyolysis, burns
• **Redistribution**   Metabolic acidosis   Hyperglycemia
• **Hypoaldosteronism**   Addison's disease   Acute renal failure
• **Drug induced**   Potassium sparing diuretics   Non-steroidal anti-inflammatory drugs   Anti-angiotensin drugs (ACEi & ARBs)
• **Genetic Causes**   Hyperkalemic periodic paralysis   Renal tubular acidosis Type 4.

There are several causes of hyperkalemia which have been enlisted in Table 37.2. True gain of potassium is often due to hemolysis, rhabdomyolysis, burns or tumour lysis. Redistribution of potassium occurs in metabolic acidosis (extracellular shift), with beta-blocker therapy and in severe insulin deficiency. Hyperkalemia is a feature of hypoaldosteronism due to Addison's disease or acute on chronic renal failure. Drugs known to cause hyperkalemia include potassium-sparing diuretics, non steroidal anti-inflammatory drugs (NSAIDs), and the angiotensin converting enzyme (ACE) inhibitors. Genetic causes of hyperkalemia are Type 4 renal tubular acidosis (RTA-4) and hyperkalemic periodic paralysis.

The clinical picture of hyperkalemia depends upon the cause. The most common scenario is of acute on chronic renal failure with fluid overload, hypertension and metabolic acidosis, which are characteristic features of uremia. Sometimes, hyperkalemia is a part of diabetic ketoacidosis. At other times, burns and crush-injuries with rhabdomyolysis are associated with hyperkalemia. Severe hyperkalemia can cause serious ventricular arrhythmias.

Table 37.3: Management of hyperkalemia
• Calcium gluconate injection
• Glucose-insulin infusion
• Nebulized salbutamol
• Oral polystyrene resin
• Hemodialysis

MANAGEMENT ISSUES

Since hyperkalemia can cause serious ventricular arrhythmias, the first priority is to protect the heart. Calcium gluconate has membrane stabilizing properties and is administered intravenously as 10 ml of 10% injection over 10 minutes. The next step is to drive potassium into the cells using 100 ml of 25% glucose with 10 units of insulin given by an infusion. Nebulized salbutamol increases the urinary excretion of potassium by increasing the Na-K-ATPase pump activity. Excess potassium in the body can be depleted by potassium-binding resin like polystyrene sulphonate administered orally. Finally, if severe hyperkalemia is associated with metabolic acidosis and fluid overload, hemodialysis is the answer (Table 37.3).

Electrocardiac Syndromes

C A S E
38

Prolonged Q-T Syndrome

CASE PRESENTATION

A 62-year old woman visited her cardiologist along with her daughter, because of two episodes of syncope in the preceding week. The fainting episodes were preceded by palpitation and associated with blurring of vision. The patient was a known case of coronary heart disease and she had sustained an anterior wall myocardial infarction ten months back. At that time, she did not receive thrombolytic therapy because of late presentation to the hospital and she had also declined coronary angiography. The patient also felt breathless on exertion and her echocardiogram showed a large anterior wall motion abnormality with an ejection fraction of 30+5%. About a month back, she underwent 24-hour Holter monitoring which showed multifocal ventricular premature beats, with short runs of ventricular tachycardia. Therefore, she was prescribed amiodarone, in addition to her usual medication which included ramipril, frusemide, aspirin, atorvastatin and isosorbide mononitrate. An initial loading dose of 1200 mg per day of amiodarone, was tapered to a maintenance dose of 400 mg daily after one week.

On examination, the patient was apprehensive and tachypneic. The pulse was fast and low in volume with a few "missed beats". The heart rate was 104 beats/min. with a BP of 110/66 mm Hg. The cardiac apical impulse was diffuse and displaced towards the axilla. The S_1 and S_2 were normal with an S_3 gallop sound in diastole. No murmur or friction rub was audible. There were bilateral basilar rales over the lung fields. An ECG was obtained (Fig. 38.1).

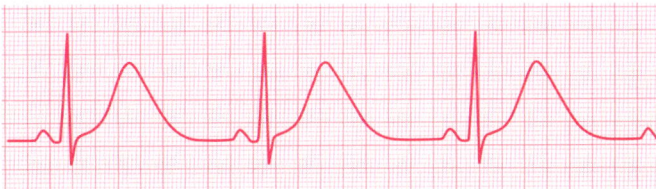

Figure 38.1: ECG showing broad T waves with prolonged Q-T interval

ECG INTERPRETATION

The ECG showed normal regular sinus rhythm. The P waves were normal in morphology and large Q waves were seen in the anterior precordial leads. The

T wave was upright, tall and broad, which occupied most of the R-R interval. The measured Q-T interval was 0.60 sec. This finding is consistent with the diagnosis of long Q-T syndrome.

The duration of the QRS complex represents ventricular depolarization time and the width of the T wave represents ventricular repolarization time. Therefore, the Q-T interval is a measure of the total duration of ventricular electrical systole. The Q-T interval is measured on the horizontal axis, from the onset of the Q wave to the termination of the T wave (not the U wave). The duration of the QRS complex, the length of the S-T segment and the width of the T wave are included in the measurement of the Q-T interval (Fig. 38.2).

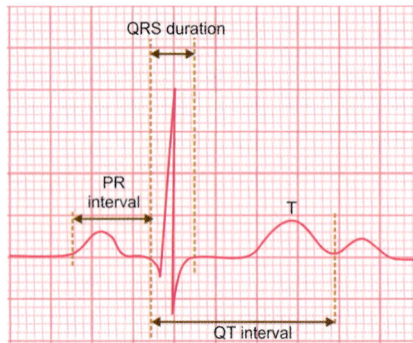

Figure 38.2 : Measurement of the Q-T interval

The upper limit of normal Q-T interval depends upon several variables, including the age, gender and the autonomic tone. It tends to be shorter in young individuals (0.44 sec) and longer in the elderly (0.45 sec). It is slightly shorter in males than in females, the upper limit being 0.43 sec in men. The Q-T interval shortens at fast heart rates and lengthens at slow heart rates. Since the Q-T interval varies with tachycardia and bradycardia, the measured Q-T interval needs to be corrected for heart rate.

The corrected Q-T interval is known as the Q-Tc interval. For heart rate correction, the Bazett's formula is generally used, where Q-Tc interval is equal to the measured Q-T interval divided by the square-root of the R-R interval. When the heart rate is 60 beats/min. and the R-R interval is 1 sec (25 x 0.04sec), the Q-Tc interval and the Q-T interval are the same. As a general rule, a Q-T interval that exceeds half of the R-R interval, is taken as a prolonged Q-T interval.

CLINICAL DISCUSSION

There are several causes of Q-T interval prolongation. These have been enlisted in Table 38.1. Congenital long Q-T syndromes may present dramatically with syncope. Indeed, congenital long Q-T syndromes are characterized by prolongation of the Q-T interval, syncope, 'seizures' and sudden death due to ventricular arrhythmias (Torsade de pointes), in apparently healthy children and young adults. Some cases of sudden infant deaths have been attributed to congenital long Q-T syndrome. Therefore, an ECG should be performed in all

Table 38.1: Causes of prolonged Q-T interval
Congenital causes
• Jervell-Lange-Neilsen syndrome (autosomal recessive with deafness)
• Romano-Ward syndrome (autosomal dominant without deafness)
Acquired causes
• Electrolyte deficiency e.g. calcium, potassium
• Antiarrhythmic drugs e.g. quinidine, amiodarone
• Coronary artery disease e.g. myocardial infarction
• Myocarditis e.g. viral myocarditis, rheumatic fever
• Intracranial event e.g. head injury, brain hemorrhage
• Bradyarrhythmias e.g. A-V block, sinus bradycardia
• Drug induced e.g. terfenadine, cisapride, olanzapine

infants on anticonvulsants for seizure prophylaxis. The prognosis and triggers of sudden cardiac death in patients with congenital long Q-T syndrome, are related to the Q-T interval and the genotype.

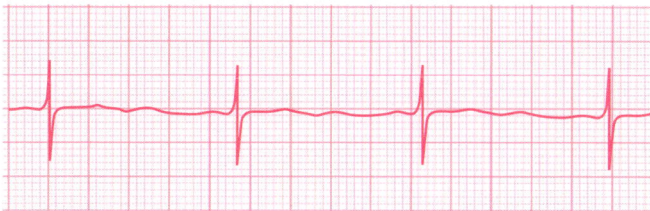

Figure 38.3 : ECG showing pseudo-prolongation of the Q-T interval

In hypokalemia, the T wave is flattened and the prominent U wave may be mistaken for the T wave. This may falsely suggest prolongation of the Q-T interval, whereas it is actually the Q-U interval. Hypokalemia therefore, cause pseudo-prolongation of the Q-T interval (Fig. 38.3). Antiarrhythmic drugs such as quinidine, procainamide and amiodarone can prolong the Q-T interval. They also cause widening of the QRS complex which, if it exceeds 25% of baseline, is an indication for withdrawing the culprit drug. Since Q-T interval prolongation predisposes to arrhythmias, this is the mechanism to explain the arrhythmia enhancing property or proarrhythmic effect of antiarrhythmic drugs. Besides antiarrhythmic agents, certain non-cardiovascular drugs can also prolong the Q-T interval. These drugs are listed in Table 38.2.

The clinical importance of Q-T interval prolongation lies in the fact that it predisposes to a typical type of polymorphic ventricular tachycardia.This tachycardia is known as "Torsade de pointes", a ballet term which literally means "torsion around a point". This term explains the morphology of the ventricular tachycardia, which consists of polymorphic QRS complexes that keep changing

Table 38.2: Drugs causing Q-T interval prolongation	
Antiarrhythmics	**Anti-infectives**
Quinidine	Erythromycin
Procainamide	Gatifloxacin
Amiodarone	Ketoconazole
Psychiatry drugs	**Miscellaneous**
Imipramine	Cisapride
Haloperidol	Terfenadine
Amitryptyline	Ketanserin

in amplitude and direction (Fig. 38.4). The polymorphic QRS complexes give the appearance of periodic torsion or twisting around the isoelectric line.

Long Q-T syndrome (LQTS) belongs to a class of congenital channelopathies, that are responsible for about 5 to 10% cases of sudden cardiac death (SCD). Other conditions belonging to this class are the Brugada syndrome and catecholaminergic ventricular tachycardia (CVT). Besides these above channelopathies, structural heart diseases responsible for SCD are hypertrophic cardiomyopathy and arrhythmogenic right ventricular dysplasia.

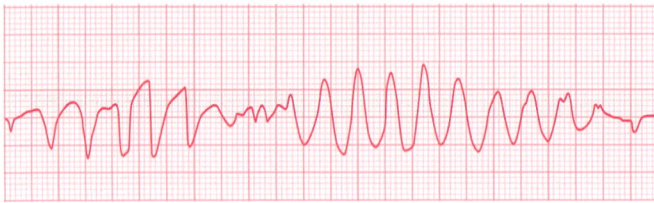

Figure 38.4: Polymorphic ventricular tachycardia ('Torsades de pointes')

MANAGEMENT ISSUES

The treatment of long Q-T syndrome depends upon the cause. When the cause is reversible, it suffices to correct the electrolyte abnormality or to withdraw the offending drug. The Q-T interval should be carefully assessed at peak plasma concentration, if multiple drugs with Q-T prolonging effect are used. In Q-T interval prolongation due to a cardiovascular or intracranial event, the underlying condition has to be managed. Since patients with congenital long Q-T syndrome are prone to syncope and sudden death due to ventricular arrhythmias, an implantable cardioverter defibrillator (ICD) is advocated.

The management of polymorphic ventricular tachycardia ("Torsades de pointes") due to long Q-T interval, is different from the management of mono-morphic ventricular tachycardia. In the acute setting, an infusion of magnesium sulphate or isoproterenol (a beta-blocker) is used. If the patient does not respond, overdrive ventricular pacing or electrical cardioversion is performed. An implantable cardioverter defibrillator (ICD) is offered to those who develop recurrent syncope, have family history of sudden cardiac death (SCD) and to survivors of cardiac arrest. To patients of congenital long QT syndrome (LQTS), cervical sympathetic ganglionectomy can be offered.

Sick Sinus Syndrome

CASE PRESENTATION

A 78-year old elderly gentleman was paid a domiciliary visit by his physician, to evaluate frequent spells of dizziness over the past 2 weeks. The patient felt light-headed when he stood up from the sitting or lying down position. Fortunately, he had never fallen down or fainted because he used a walking aid and was regularly looked after by a personal attendant. There was no history of breathlessness, chest pain or palpitation. The patient was hypertensive for over 40 years and took his medicines regularly. There was no past history of myocardial infarction or paralytic stroke. The only time he was hospitalized was for prostate surgery five years back. The patient's family members had also noticed recent mental confusion and lapses in his memory.

On examination, the patient was conscious and cooperative but somewhat confused. The pulse was irregular, good in volume, at a rate of 48 to 52 beats/min. The dorsalis pedis pulsations were diminished on both sides and a bruit was audible over the left carotid artery. The BP was 160/82 mm Hg in the supine position and 150/74 mm Hg while standing. The JVP was not raised and there was no pitting edema over the ankles. The S_1 was normal and A_2 was loud; no S_3 or S_4 sound was audible. A short harsh systolic murmur was heard over the upper parasternal area. A different blowing pansystolic murmur was heard over the cardiac apex, that radiated towards the axilla. Breath sounds were vesicular, without any crepitations. An ECG was obtained (Fig. 39.1). At the time of prostate surgery, an ECHO had shown mild concentric left ventricular hypertrophy with an ejection fraction of 52% and no regional wall motion abnormality. CT scan of the head at the same time showed periventricular lacunar infarcts and changes of diffuse cerebral atrophy.

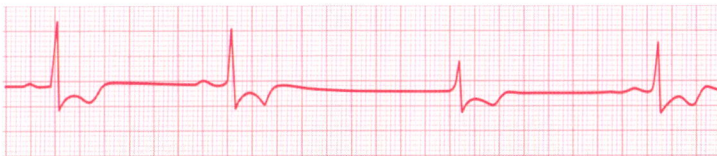

Figure 39.1: ECG showing sinus bradycardia, asystole and junctional escape

ECG INTERPRETATION

The ECG showed sinus bradycardia at a rate of 50 beats/min., with short periods of asystole. At times the R-R interval was twice the usual R-R interval, suggesting 2:1 sino-atrial exit block (S-A block). At other times, the period of asystole was followed by a delayed beat without a preceding P wave, consistent with a junctional escape beat. This constellation of ECG findings which includes sinus bradycardia, S-A block and junctional escape, is consistent with the diagnosis of sinus node dysfunction, the so called sick sinus syndrome (Table 39.1).

Table 39.1: ECG findings in sick sinus syndrome
• Sinus bradycardia
• Sino-atrial exit block
• Slow atrial fibrillation
• Junctional escape rhythm

The sick sinus syndrome usually presents with bradyarrhythmias such as those mentioned above. At times the indications of sinus node dysfunction are an inadequate tachycardia with sympathomimetic drugs, excessive sensitivity to beta-blocker drugs and atropine resistant bradycardia. At other times, there may be atrial fibrillation with slow ventricular response or a junctional rhythm. The coexistence of fast and slow cardiac rhythms constitutes the so called "tachy-brady" syndrome.

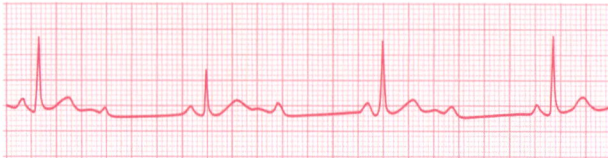

Figure 39.2: ECG showing 2:1 atrio-ventricular (A-V) block

In a pause due to 2:1 sino-atrial (S-A) exit block, the entire P-QRS-T complex is missing, since neither atrial nor ventricular activation occurs. By contrast in 2:1 atrio-ventricular (A-V) block, the P wave is inscribed normally but not followed by a QRS complex (Fig. 39.2). S-A block may coexist with A-V block and even left bundle branch block, if fibrocalcerous degeneration involves the entire conduction system. Quite often, sinus node dysfunction is suspected clinically but difficult to prove because the ECG is normal and Holter monitoring does not show up the arrhythmia, during the period of observation. A prolonged sinus node recovery time (SNRT) and sino-atrial conduction time (SACT) on electrophysiological studies (EPS) is then taken as a diagnostic criteria for sick sinus syndrome (SSS).

CLINICAL DISCUSSION

The "sick sinus syndrome" (SSS) is a clinical condition caused by a diseased sinus node, which fails to produce or successfully conduct a sufficient number of cardiac impulses. It is observed in elderly patients and is believed to be caused by a degenerative condition like amyloidosis or infiltration of the atrium by a fibro-calcerous process. Certain cardiovascular drugs notably beta-blockers (atenolol, metoprolol), calcium-blockers (verapamil, diltiazem) and digoxin may also cause sinus node dysfunction, which is reversible after discontinuation of therapy.

Table 39.2: Symptoms of sick sinus syndrome
• Dizziness and syncope
• Dyspnea and fatigue
• Palpitation and angina
• Confusion and dementia

The most frequent symptoms of sick sinus syndrome are dizziness, mental confusion and fainting attacks (Table 39.2). Spells of dizziness and syncope in sick sinus syndrome are due to transient ventricular asystole, causing a precipitous decline in stroke volume and cerebral perfusion. Such episodes are known as Stokes-Adams attacks. Besides SSS, other causes of Stokes-Adam's attacks are advanced atrio-ventricular block, malignant ventricular arrhythmias, carotid sinus hypersensitivity and subclavian steal syndrome (Table 39.3).

Table 39.3: Causes of Stokes Adams Attacks
• Advanced atrio-ventricular block
• Serious ventricular arrhythmias
• Carotid sinus hypersensitivity
• Subclavian steal syndrome
• Sick sinus syndrome

Since patients are in the advanced age group, many of them have had a cerebrovascular accident or a prior myocardial infarction. They may also complain of dyspnea and fatigue due to heart failure. Palpitation and angina pectoris may occur due to tachyarrhythmias or associated coronary artery disease. Dizziness and syncope in an elderly patient may be multifactorial. Even those with documented sick sinus syndrome may additionally have volume depletion, electrolyte imbalance or hypoglycemia. They may have orthostatic hypotension due to autonomic failure or vertebro-basilar insufficiency. Still others may have cardiac outflow obstruction due to aortic sclerosis or ventricular arrhythmias due to an old myocardial scar or heart failure. Therefore, a detailed evaluation of these patients is warranted.

MANAGEMENT ISSUES

Drugs that can increase the rate of discharge from the sinus node such as sympathomimetic (adrenaline) and vagolytic (atropine) drugs, can only temporarily increase the heart rate. Permanent pacemaker implantation (PPI) is the definitive form of treatment, particularly if the symptoms are severe and disabling. Dual-chamber pacemakers are more physiological and carry a lower risk of atrial fibrillation and stroke. They also have a distinct advantage over single-chamber pacing if there is coexistent A-V nodal disease or bundle branch block. Pacemaker implantation makes it possible to use antiarrhythmic drugs to treat tachyarrhythmias, which otherwise would have caused severe bradycardia.

Early Repolarization Syndrome

A 29-year old well-built man of African origin, sought an appointment with the cardiologist, for opinion on an abnormal ECG. The ECG was performed as part of routine pre-employment medical evaluation. The man vehemently denied complaints of fatigue, breathlessness, chest pain, palpitation or syncope. He had been actively involved in competitive sports during his college days and still played tennis on week-ends. The man did not smoke or take alcohol, but was fond of calorie-dense food. He did not suffer from diabetes or hypertension and had never got a serum lipid analysis done. There was no family history of coronary heart disease or of cerebrovascular accident.

On examination, the man was of stocky built, with a muscular physique. His body mass index (BMI) was 28 kg/m². He was fully conscious, comfortable and cheerful. There was no anemia, cyanosis, icterus or edema. The trachea was central, thyroid gland was not palpable and the JVP was not raised. The pulse rate was 58-62 beats/min. with a normal pulse volume and no special character. The BP was 120/80 mm Hg over the right arm. The precordium was unremarkable, with a normally located apex beat. The S$_1$ and S$_2$ were normal without any gallop sound. No murmur or pericardial friction rub was audible. The breath sounds were vesicular without any audible rhonchi or crepitations. A fresh ECG was performed in the cardiologist's office (Fig. 40.1).

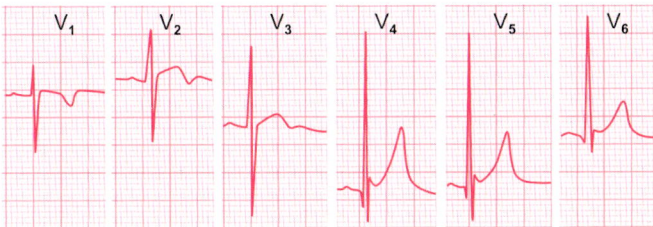

Figure 40.1: ECG showing features of early repolarization syndrome

ECG INTERPRETATION

The ECG showed tall R waves in the lateral precordial leads, preceded by narrow Q waves. The S-T segment was elevated concave upwards, with an initial slur on the S-T segment (J wave). The T waves were upright, tall and symmetrical in the lateral leads, with prominent U waves in the mid-precordial leads. These findings are consistent with the diagnosis of early repolarization syndrome (Table 40.1). Since early repolarization is frequently observed in healthy athletic persons, this entity is also known as the "athlete's heart".

There are several causes of S-T segment elevation (Table 40.2), of which acute myocardial infarction is the leading cause. The S-T segment elevation of early repolarization, can simulate the injury pattern of acute myocardial infarction. However, there are several classical differentiating features:

- S-T segment elevation is concave upwards in lead V_6
- Ratio of S-T elevation : T wave height is below 0.25
- There is no reciprocal S-T depression in other leads
- ECG changes do not evolve as in case of infarction
- ECHO does not show abnormal regional wall motion
- Serial level of cardiac enzyme titers are not increased.

Table 40.1: ECG features of early repolarization syndrome

- Tall R wave in lead V_6
- Narrow and deep Q wave
- Concave S-T segment elevation
- Initial J wave on the S-T segment
- Upright and tall symmetrical T wave

CLINICAL DISCUSSION

The "early repolarization" variant is an alarming electrocardiographic entity, which presents with S-T segment elevation. It represents early repolarization of a portion of the ventricle, before the entire myocardium has been depolarized. There is an early uptake of the S-T segment, before the descending limb of the R wave has reached the baseline. This causes an initial slur on the S-T segment, known as the J wave. The S-T segment is elevated and concave upwards. There is an associated increased amplitude of the R wave. The T wave is also tall, but the ratio of S-T segment elevation to T wave height is less than 0.25. Interestingly, the degree of S-T elevation and T wave height may vary on a day-to-day basis and the S-T segment may normalize after exercise. Besides the features already mentioned, other characteristics of this syndrome are sinus bradycardia with sinus arrhythmia, voltage criteria of left ventricular hypertrophy and persistent juvenile pattern of T wave inversion in leads V_1 to V_3.

Table 40.2: Causes of S-T segment elevation

Coronary artery disease

- Myocardial infarction
- Prinzmetal's angina
- Dressler's syndrome
- Ventricular aneurysm

Non-coronary disease

- Acute pericarditis
- Pulmonary embolism
- Early repolarization
- Brugada syndrome

Early repolarization is more frequently observed among young athletic males of Africo-Carribean descent. They are healthy subjects who are free of symptoms and their clinical examination is entirely normal. Acute viral pericarditis also presents with concave-upwards S-T segment elevation but sinus tachycardia is almost invariably present. Moreover, patients of acute pericarditis have a preceding flu-like illness, they present with chest pain and there is an audible pericardial rub.

MANAGEMENT ISSUES

Individuals who have features of early reploarization on the ECG, are healthy asymptomatic subjects without any objective evidence of organic heart disease. Therefore, no specific treatment apart from reassurance is advocated. However, lack of awareness about this entity may lead to unnecessary investigations including stress-testing, myocardial perfusion imaging and coronary angiography.

41

Brugada Syndrome

CASE PRESENTATION

A 28-year old man was asked to see a cardiologist by a general physician, for expert opinion on an abnormal ECG. The ECG had been performed by the physician empanelled with an insurance company, as part of the pre-insurance medical check-up. The man clearly denied any history of chest pain, dyspnea, palpitation or syncope. He was physically very active and undertook a brisk walk for 40 minutes, on most days of the week. He had also been a regular member of his school and college cricket teams. The man smoked about 5 cigarettes a day and consumed about 1 litre of beer on week-ends. His blood pressure and blood sugar levels were normal but his lipid profile showed an elevated LDL value. One of his cousin brothers had died of cardiac arrest, at the age of 32 years.

On examination, the man was well built and had a healthy appearance with a body mass index (BMI) of 26 kg/m². He was conscious, comfortable and cooperative during examination. There was no anemia, cyanosis, jaundice or ankle edema. The pulse rate was 72 beats/min.; pulse was fair in volume and had no special character. The BP in the right arm was 120/80 mm Hg. The precordium was unremarkable and the cardiac apex beat was normally located. The S_1 and S_2 were normal and no S_3 or S_4 sound was heard. No murmur or pericardial friction rub was audible. The breath sounds were normal and no rhonchi or crepts were heard over the lung fields. A fresh ECG was obtained in the office of the cardiologist (Fig. 41.1).

ECG INTERPRETATION

The ECG showed a triphasic rSR′ pattern in lead V_1, which was 0.10 second in duration. Additionally, there was a "tent-like" coved S-T segment elevation of 0.2 mV with large inverted T waves (Table 41.1). These findings are consistent with the diagnosis of Brugada syndrome. Three types of S-T segment elevation are described in Brugada syndrome, depending upon the ventricular repolarization pattern.

- Type 1: "Tent-like" coved S-T segment, elevation >0.2 mV, negative T wave
- Type 2: "Saddle-back like" S-T segment, elevation >0.1 mV, positive T wave
- Type 3: "Saddle-back like" S-T segment, elevation <0.1 mV, positive T wave.

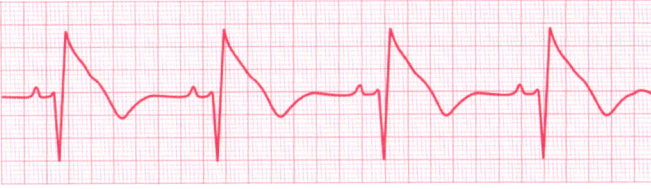

Figure 41.1: ECG showing features of the Brugada syndrome.

Table 41.1: ECG Features of Brugada Syndrome
• rSR' pattern in lead V_1
• rSR' duration < 0.12 sec
• Large and inverted T wave
• Coved S-T segment elevation

Besides Brugada syndrome, other causes of S-T segment elevation in lead V_1 are right ventricular infarction, acute pulmonary embolism and arrhythmogenic right ventricular dysplasia (Table 41.2). The rSR pattern in lead V_1 observed in case of Brugada syndrome, superficially resembles right branch block (RBBB). But unlike in RBBB, the ventricular complex is not more than 0.12 sec wide and there are no broad S waves in lead L_1 and V_6. The characteristic ECG abnormalities observed in Brugada syndrome may only be transient and not observed constantly. These may become exaggerated or unmasked after drug challenge with antiarrhythmic agents such as flecainide and procainamide.

Table 41.2 : Causes of S-T segment elevation in lead V_1
• Brugada syndrome
• Right ventricular infarction
• Acute pulmonary embolism
• Arrhythmogenic RV dysplasia.

CLINICAL DISCUSSION

The Brugada syndrome is a rare but striking electrocardiographic abnormality. It is believed to be a genetic disorder of sodium transport, across ion channels located in the right ventricle. This produces an abnormal pattern of right ventricular depolarization. Patients who have this abnormality are prone to develop sudden syncope because of malignant ventricular tachycardia or even cardiac arrest due to ventricular fibrillation. The genetic defect underlying Brugada syndrome may exist in more than one family member and form the basis of familial ventricular arrhythmias. The disorder is transmitted down subsequent generations by autosomal dominant inheritance.

Brugada syndrome belongs to a class of congenital channelopathies which are responsible for nearly 5 to 10% cases of sudden cardiac death (SCD). Other members of this class are long Q-T syndrome (LQTS) and catecholaminergic ventricular tachycardia (CVT), as given in Table 41.3. Besides these channelopathies, congenital structural heart diseases responsible for SCD are hypertrophic cardiomyopathy and arrhythmogenic right ventricular dysplasia.

Table 41.3: Congenital channelopathies

- Brugada syndrome
- Long Q-T syndrome
- Catecholaminergic VT*
  (*ventricular tachycardia)

MANAGEMENT ISSUES

There is no specific treatment of the underlying disorder in Brugada syndrome. However, insertion of an automatic implantable cardioverter defibrillator (AICD) may be considered in those patients with history of recurrent syncope, after cardiac resuscitation from ventricular fibrillation, or if there is history of sudden cardiac death in a family member.

CASE

42

WPW Syndrome

CASE PRESENTATION

A 24-year old unmarried female arrived at the emergency-room, with the complaints of palpitation and light-headedness for the last 15 minutes. She drove herself to the hospital and admitted that she felt dizzy while driving. The patient also gave history of several such episodes in the past. At times, she was able to abort the attack by splashing cold water on her face, or by applying firm pressure over the eyes. At other times, she had to rush to the hospital, as on that day. During the "machine-like" sensation over the chest, she never experienced any chest pain or difficulty in breathing. However, after the palpitation stopped, she would pass a large volume of urine. The onset of these episodes was unrelated to physical exercise, emotional stress or to the intake of any particular food or beverage. There was no history of tremor, heat-intolerance, undue fatigue or significant weight-loss.

On examination, the patient was apprehensive but not tachypneic. The extremities were not cold but her palms were sweaty. The pulse rate was extremely rapid and exceeded 150 beats/min, although it could not be counted accurately. The BP was 91/64 mm Hg over the right arm and she was apyrexial. There were no signs of congestive heart failure. There was no goitre, bruit over the thyroid gland or any clinical sign of Grave's disease. The precordium was normal and the apex beat was normally located. There was extreme tachycardia and the character of S_1 and S_2 could not be appreciated. The attending doctor performed right carotid sinus massage which resulted in sudden termination of the patient's symptoms and a remarkable change in her heart rate. An ECG was obtained afterwards (Fig. 42.1).

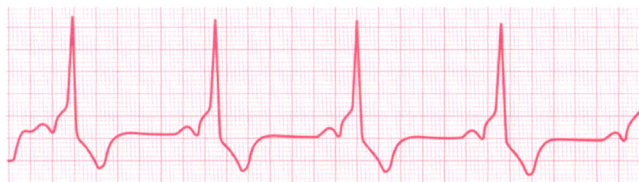

Figure 42.1: ECG showing features of the WPW Syndrome

ECG INTERPRETATION

The ECG showed normal P waves with a P-R interval of 0.08 sec. The width of the QRS complex was 0.12 sec with a notch on the ascending limb of the R wave. There was depression of the S-T segment with inversion of the T wave. These findings are consistent with the diagnosis of WPW syndrome. The Wolff-Parkinson-White (WPW) Syndrome is a distinct electrocardiographic entity wherein an accessory pathway, the bundle of Kent, directly connects the atrial myocardium to the ventricular myocardium, bypassing the A-V node (Fig. 42.2). This produces abnormalities of the QRS complex, P-R interval, S-T segment and the T wave.

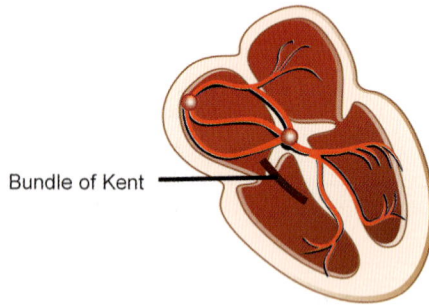

Figure 42.2: Diagram to illustrate the Bundle of Kent

The P-R interval is short because ventricular depolarization through the accessory pathway, bypasses the normal conduction delay at the A-V node. The notch on the ascending limb of R wave is the delta wave. It indicates pre-excitation of the ventricle through the accessory pathway, before depolarization of the entire ventricle by the normal conduction system. The QRS complex is wide because it is a fusion beat, which is the sum of ventricular prexcitation and normal ventricular depolarization. The S-T segment and T wave inversion are repolarization abnormalities, secondary to the abnormal pattern of ventricular depolarization (Fig. 42.3).

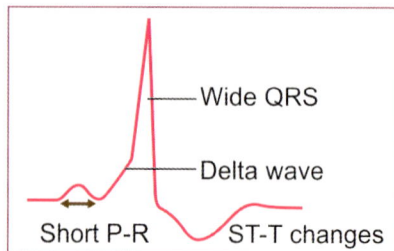

Figure 42.3: ECG in case of WPW syndrome

Three types of QRS configuration are described in the WPW syndrome, depending upon the direction of the accessory pathway.

- Type A (left septal connection) produces upright QRS complexes in all the precordial leads. It resembles right bundle branch block or true posterior wall myocardial infarction.
- Type B (right-sided connection) has negative QRS complexes in V_1 and positive complexes in lead V_6. It resembles left bundle branch block or left ventricular hypertrophy.
- Type C (left lateral connection) has positive QRS complexes in lead V_1 and negative complexes in lead V_6. It resembles right ventricular hypertrophy.

CLINICAL DISCUSSION

The standardized nomenclature of pre-excitation syndromes uses the term "tract" for pathways that insert into specialized conduction tissue and "connection" for pathways that enter the general myocardium. The Wolff-Parkinson-White (WPW) syndrome involves an atrio-ventricular connection (Kent bundle). Lown-Ganong-Levine (LGL) syndrome involves an atrio-fascicular bypass tract (James bundle) (Fig. 42.4). Mahaim fibers constitute a fasciculo-ventricular connection.

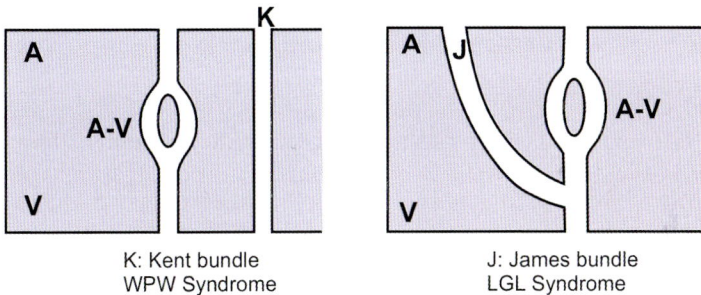

K: Kent bundle
WPW Syndrome

J: James bundle
LGL Syndrome

Figure 42.4: Diagram to illustrate the various pre-excitation syndromes
A: Atrium; V: Ventricle; A-V: Atrio-ventricular

The WPW syndrome is a masquerader of several other cardiac conditions:
- The delta wave as separate from the R wave can mimic bundle branch block.
- The dominant R wave in lead V_1 may resemble right ventricular hypertrophy.
- Negative delta wave with S-T segment depression and T wave inversion, may appear as myocardial infarction.
- Antidromic A-V re-entrant tachycardia conducted anterogradely through the accessory pathway may be mistaken for ventricular tachycardia.

The clinical importance of the WPW syndrome lies in the fact that it predisposes to paroxysmal atrial tachycardia, since the bypass tract forms a re-entrant circuit with the regular conduction pathway. Paroxysmal atrial tachycardia (PAT) in the presence of WPW syndrome needs to be differentiated from a PAT without an accessory pathway, since the management is somewhat different.

MANAGEMENT ISSUES

Presence of the WPW syndrome predisposes an individual to paroxysmal supraventricular tachycardia (PSVT), wherein the bypass tract constitutes a re-entrant circuit along with the normal conduction pathway. In almost 90% patients, conduction proceeds anterogradely down the A-V node and returns retrogradely through the accessory pathway to the atrium. This is known as orthodromic tachycardia and here the QRS complex is narrow. This arrhythmia responds to vagal manoeuvres and to drugs used in the treatment of A-V nodal re-entrant tachycardia (AVNRT). These drugs include verapamil, diltiazem, digitalis and adenosine.

In less than 10% patients, anterograde conduction proceeds down the accessory pathway and returns retrogradely through the normal A-V nodal pathway to the atrium. This is known as antidromic tachycardia and here the QRS complex is wide and demonstrates the WPW syndrome. This arrhythmia does not respond to vagal manoeuvres, but only to cardioversion with DC shock or to antiarrhythmic drugs that block the accessory pathway such as amiodarone.

Cardiac Arrhythmias

CASE
43

Supraventricular Tachycardia

CASE PRESENTATION

A 36-year old woman had been experiencing episodes of "fluttering" sensation in the chest, since two years. The episodes were described as a "machine-like" feeling over the precordium, that was not accompanied by chest pain or shortness of breath. During these episodes she did feel dizzy, but she never lost her consciousness. Once the episode was over, she would pass urine frequently. Her episodes were unrelated to physical exertion, food intake or to mental stress. At times she was able to abort the attack on her own, either by splashing cold water on her face or by applying firm pressure over her eyes. At other times, she had to visit a cardiologist who either performed carotid sinus massage or administered intravenous diltiazem. Initially, episodes would occur only once in a month or two but recently, their frequency had increased significantly. Therefore, although she was prescribed verapamil 120 mg twice a day which she took regularly, the patient was advised to undergo electrophysiological studies (EPS).

On examination, the patient was apprehensive but not tachypneic or in any distress. The heart rate exceeded 150 beats/min., with a BP of 96/70 mm Hg and she was afebrile. The JVP was not raised and there was no edema over the ankles. There was no tremor over fingers, thyromegaly or eye prominence to suggest thyrotoxicosis. The precordium was hyperkinetic in nature, with a normally located apex beat. On auscultation, S_3 or S_4 sound could not be appreciated because of extreme tachycardia, but no murmur or friction rub was audible. Breath sounds were vesicular without any rhonchi or crepts. A long-strip ECG recording of lead L_{II} was obtained (Fig. 43.1).

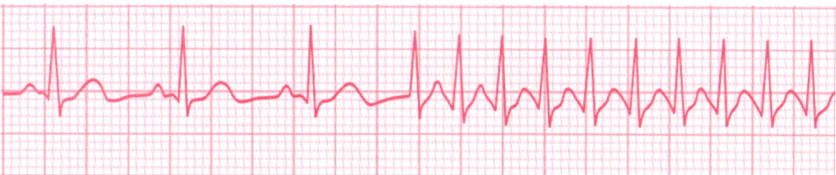

Figure 43.1: ECG showing abrupt onset of narrow QRS tachycardia

ECG INTERPRETATION

The ECG showed an abrupt onset of regular tachycardia at a rate exceeding 150 beats/min., with an R-R interval of less than 10mm. The QRS complexes were narrow and the P or T waves were not visible. These findings are consistent with the diagnosis of paroxysmal supraventricular tachycardia (PSVT).

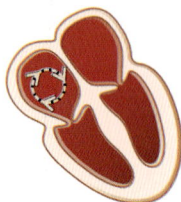

Figure 43.2: Diagram to illustrate circus movement in a closed re-entrant circuit

Supraventricular tachycardia is most often (in 90% cases) based on repetitive circus movement of impulses in a closed re-entrant circuit (re-entrant tachycardia). In 50% cases, the circuit is composed of two pathways within the atrioventricular node (AV nodal reentrant tachycardia-AVNRT). In 40% cases, the circuit consists of an AV nodal pathway and an accessory bypass tract along its side (AV re-entrant tachycardia-AVRT). An atrial impulse first passes anterogradely down one of the two pathways, the other pathway being in the refractory period. The impulses then returns retrogradely through the other pathway, which has by now recovered its conductivity. In this way, repetitive circulation of impulses occurs, to produce a sustained atrial tachycardia (Fig. 43.2). Least often (in about 10% cases), supraventricular tachycardia is due to rapid discharge of impulses from an ectopic atrial focus (ectopic atrial tachycardia).

The heart rate in paroxysmal atrial tachycardia is 150 to 200 beats per minute, if a re-entrant circuit is involved. It tends to be slower in ectopic atrial tachycardia (120 to 150 beats/min), as the A-V node cannot conduct more than 150 atrial impulses per minute. The heart rate can exceed a rate of 200 beats/min, if an accessory bypass tract is involved, as in case of WPW syndrome. This is because in WPW syndrome, the impulses can bypass the decremental influence of the A-V node, by travelling down the accessory pathway. An atrial tachycardia arising

Table 43.1: Differences between ectopic and re-entrant atrial tachycardia		
	Ectopic tachycardia	**Re-entrant tachycardia**
Heart rate	120-150/min	More than 150/min
Onset and offset	Gradual	Sudden
P wave	Ectopic, visible	Inverted, Rarely visible
A-V block	Can coexist	Never, 1:1 conduction
Effect of vagal manoeuvre	Slowing	Termination
Past history	Not significant	Previous episodes
Organic heart disease	May be present	Generally absent

from an ectopic focus can be differentiated from a tachycardia due to a re-entrant mechanism, by certain subtle features (Table 43.1).

Most often, a supraventricular tachycardia is characterized by narrow QRS complexes, due to synchronized ventricular activation through the specialized His bundle conduction system. Occasionally, the supraventricular impulses find one

Table 43.2: Differences between ventricular tachycardia and aberrant ventricular conduction		
	Ventricular tachycardia	**SVT with aberrancy**
Regularity of rhythm	Slightly irregular	Clock-like regularity
P waves	Not seen	May be seen
P-QRS relationship	Unrelated	Related
QRS width	> 0.14 sec	0.12-0.14 sec
QRS morphology	Bizarre	Triphasic
QRS in V_1 to V_6	rS in V_1 to V_6	RsR' in V_1; Rs in V_6
R-R' height	R > R'	R' > R
QRS axis	Leftward	Normal
Capture/fusion beats	May be seen	Not seen
Hemodynamics	Compromised	Stable
Organic heart disease	Often present	Often absent
Response to carotid massage	No response	Termination

of the two bundle branches refractory to conduction. In that case, the impulses are conducted only through the other bundle branch, producing a situation of aberrant ventricular conduction. This needs to be differentiated from a wide QRS ventricular tachycardia. The differences between ventricular tachycardia and supraventricular tachycardia with aberrant ventricular conduction are given in Table 43.2.

CLINICAL DISCUSSION

Paroxysmal re-entrant atrial tachycardia is most often based on a reciprocal mechanism involving a bypass tract or a dual intranodal pathway. Episodes of atrial tachycardia are one of the manifestations of pre-excitation (WPW syndrome). In the absence of WPW syndrome, paroxysmal atrial tachycardia (PAT) is generally not associated with organic heart disease. If properly managed, PAT does not alter life-expectancy and carries an excellent prognosis. PAT coexisting with the WPW syndrome carries a poorer prognosis, because of the risk of degeneration into ventricular tachycardia. A paroxysm of atrial tachycardia in the presence of an underlying WPW syndrome is suggested, if it meets one of the following criteria:

• ECG during sinus rhythm shows short P-R interval and wide QRS complex
• The ventricular rate exceeds 200 beats/minute, indicating the absence of physiological A-V block
• Inverted P waves are observed indicating retrograde atrial activation.

Symptoms due to atrial tachycardia depend upon the atrial rate, the duration of the tachycardia and the presence of heart disease. A fast atrial tachycardia causes palpitation and neck pulsations. Angina pectoris may occur due to increased myocardial oxygen demand and reduced coronary filling time. Prolonged atrial tachycardia can cause dizziness or syncope due to decline in cardiac output (shortened ventricular filling time) and loss of atrial contribution to ventricular filling. Termination of the tachycardia is often followed by polyuria due to the release of atrial natriuretic peptide (ANP) by the stretching of atrial myocardium.

MANAGEMENT ISSUES

The first step in the management of supraventricular tachycardia is to attempt vagal stimulation, to block the atrio-ventricular (AV) node. Vagal manoeuvres include carotid sinus massage, supraorbital pressure, Valsalva manoeuvre and splashing ice-cold water on the face (Table 43.3). Before commencing carotid sinus massage, the carotid artery should be auscultated for a bruit. If a bruit is present, carotid massage should not be performed on that side, or else an embolus may dislodge from the plaque. Massage should be done on one side at a time and not simultaneously on both sides. If vagal manoeuvres fail to abort the tachycardia, a drug to block the A-V node is administered intravenously. Drugs that are effective include adenosine, diltiazem and amiodarone. After restoration of sinus rhythm, oral diltiazem, verapamil, amiodarone or a beta-blocker such as metoprolol is prescribed to prevent recurrence.

Table 43.3: Management of supraventricular tachycardia
PSVT with nodal re-entry
• Vagal manoeuvres
• Adenosine, diltiazem
PSVT with bypass tract
• Amiodarone therapy
• Radiofrequency ablation

The management of paroxysmal atrial tachycardia in the presence of WPW syndrome, is somewhat different. Vagal manoeuvres are useful, only if anterograde conduction proceeds through the A-V node. Digitalis is contraindicated as it enhances conduction down the accessory pathway and may precipitate ventricular fibrillation. Diltiazem and metoprolol reduce the tolerance to the high ventricular rate and can precipitate congestive heart failure. Amiodarone is the antiarrhythmic agent of choice for the long-term treatment and prevention of arrhythmias associated with the WPW syndrome (Table 43.3).

The availability of sophisticated electrophysiological studies (EPS) to identify and locate bypass tracts and the development of latest ablative techniques, have revolutionized the management of WPW syndrome. For ablation of the bypass tract, high-frequency AC current is delivered through a thermister tipped catheter, which leads to localized heat coagulation. Radiofrequency ablation (RFA) of the bypass tract can be offered to patients who report recurrent and frequent symptomatic episodes of PAT which are refractory to drug therapy or those that cause hemodynamic compromise.

CASE PRESENTATION

A 42-year old woman presented with the complaints of palpitation and extreme fatigue. She denied history of chest pain or dizziness, but she felt tired and breathless after routine activities. During the preceding 6 months, she had unintentionally lost 4 to 5 kg of weight, despite having a good appetite. There was no history of excessive thirst or frequent urination, but she passed 3 to 4 semiformed stools everyday. The patient felt particularly uncomfortable during the summer months when her restlessness, fatigue and palpitations increased considerably. There was no history of prolonged febrile illness with joint pains during her childhood and she had never received monthly shots of penicillin. The patient was married since 16 years and had two sons who were 13 and 9 years of age. Both of them were born after normal delivery and were in good health.

On examination, the patient was restless, anxious and tachypneic. Her extremities were warm and her palms were dry. There was no anemia, cyanosis, jaundice or ankle edema. The pulse was fast, irregular and of good volume, with a pulse rate of 90 to 100 beats/min. The heart rate by auscultation was 110 to 120 beats/min, with a BP of 144/92 mm Hg over the right arm. Her temperature was 99.2⁰F and the respiratory rate was 24/min. There was tremor over her outstretched hand and the eye-balls were prominent with lid-retraction. The JVP was not raised and there were no palpable lymph-nodes, but the thyroid gland was diffusely enlarged. The goiter was not tender, but a bruit was audible. The precordium was hyperkinetic with a forceful apical impulse. The S_1 was variable in intensity with a loud S_2. No murmur or gallop sound was audible. A long-strip ECG recording of lead L_{II} was recorded (Fig. 44.1).

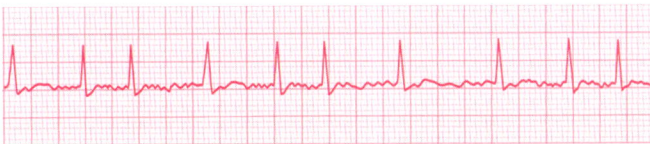

Figure 44.1: ECG showing irregular rhythm with fine fibrillatory waves

ECG INTERPRETATION

The ECG showed a fast irregular rhythm, with a variable R-R interval. The QRS complexes were narrow, but no P waves were visible. Instead, there were fine fibrillatory waves between the QRS complexes. These findings are consistent with the diagnosis of atrial fibrillation (AF). Atrial fibrillation is a grossly irregular fast rhythm produced by functional fractionation of the atria into numerous tissue islets, in various stages of excitation and recovery. Consequently, atrial activation is chaotic and ineffectual in causing atrial contraction (Fig. 44.2). Although 400 to 500 fibrillatory impulses reach the A-V node per minute, only 100 to 150 of them succeed in eliciting a ventricular response, while others are blocked in the A-V node. The random activation of the ventricles produces a grossly irregular ventricular rhythm.

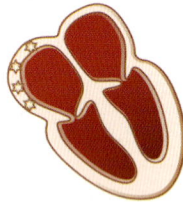

Figure 44.2: Diagram to illustrate atrial islets with chaotic atrial activation

The hallmark of atrial fibrillation is the absence of discrete P waves. Instead, there are numerous, small, irregular fibrillatory waves (f waves) that are difficult to identify individually but produce a ragged baseline. In long-standing atrial fibrillation, these undulations are minimal and produce a nearly flat baseline. As mentioned, the ventricular rate is grossly irregular and varies from 100 to 150 beats per minute. Atrial fibrillation can be differentiated from atrial flutter by the absence of P waves and an irregular ventricular rate (Table 44.1). At times, precise differentiation between the two may be difficult and the rhythm is then known as "flutter-fibrillation", "coarse fibrillation" or "impure flutter".

Table 44.1: Differences between atrial flutter and atrial fibrillation		
	Atrial flutter	**Atrial fibrillation**
Atrial rate	220-350 beats/min	Over 350 beats/min
Ventricular rate	Regular. Half to one fourth of atrial rate	Variable. No relation to atrial rate
Atrial activity	Flutter (F) waves Saw-toothed baseline	Fibrillatory (f) waves Ragged baseline
Ventricular activity	Constant R-R interval	Variable R-R interval

In atrial fibrillation, the ventricular rate generally varies from 100 to 150 beats per minute. Faster rates are observed in children, patients of thyrotoxicosis and in the presence of WPW syndrome. Slower rates are observed during drug treatment with beta-blockers (propranolol, atenolol) or calcium-blockers (verapamil, diltiazem), as these drugs block the A-V node. Elderly patients with A-V nodal disease may also manifest slow atrial fibrillation. Regularization of the ventricular rate in a patient on digitalis for atrial fibrillation, indicates the onset of junctional tachycardia and is a manifestation of digitalis toxicity.

CLINICAL DISCUSSION

Atrial fibrillation (AF) can be classified into three groups. In paroxysmal AF, discrete episodes are self-terminating and last less than 48 hours. In persistent AF, fibrillation continues unabated for atleast 7 days, but can be converted to sinus rhythm by electrical or chemical cardioversion. In permanent AF, fibrillation continues indefinitely and conversion to sinus rhythm is not possible. Atrial fibrillation can occur in virtually any form of heart disease. Common causes of atrial fibrillation are given in Table 44.2.

Table 44.2: Causes of atrial fibrillation
Persistent atrial fibrillation
• Dilated cardiomyopathy
• Constrictive pericarditis
• Cardiac trauma/surgery
• Hypertensive heart disease
• Valvular heart disease (MS)
• Coronary artery disease (MI)
• Congenital heart disease (ASD).
Paroxysmal atrial fibrillation
• Thyrotoxicosis
• WPW syndrome
• Sick sinus syndrome
• Lone atrial fibrillation
• Acute alcoholic intoxication
• Pulmonary thrombo-embolism.

The symptoms of AF depend upon the ventricular rate, the nature and severity of underlying heart disease and the effectiveness of treatment. Palpitation is due to fast heart rate while syncope is caused by reduced cerebral perfusion. Angina may occur because of increased myocardial oxygen demand as well as shortened coronary filling time due to tachycardia. Dyspnea is due to pulmonary congestion, secondary to loss of atrial contribution to ventricular filling. Sometimes, regional ischemia in the form of limb gangrene, hemiparesis or blindness may occur because of systemic embolization from a left atrial thrombus.

Atrial fibrillation can be recognized clinically by several subtle signs. The pulse is irregularly irregular, with the pulse rate on palpation being less than the heart rate on auscultation (pulse deficit). The *a* waves are not observed in the neck veins. There is a beat-to-beat variability in the pulse pressure as well as the intensity of first heart sound, because of a variable ventricular diastolic filling period.

MANAGEMENT ISSUES

The treatment of atrial fibrillation (AF) is governed by the patient's symptoms and hemodynamic status. In the majority of patients, long-term rate control along with oral anticoagulation, is a reasonable therapeutic strategy. Drugs that prolong the refractory period of the atrio-ventricular (AV) node such as digoxin, diltiazem and metoprolol are effective for rate control in persistent AF. In patients of paroxysmal AF with infrequent episodes, a "pill in the pocket" (taken when symptomatic) strategy is preferable. Drugs used for this purpose are amiodarone, sotalol, flecainide and propafenone.

Long-standing atrial fibrillation produces stasis of blood in the left atrium and promotes the development of thrombi in the atrial cavity and the atrial appendage. Dislodged fragments of these thrombi can enter the systemic circulation as emboli and settle down in any arterial territory. Anti-coagulants such as caumarin and warfarin are required for long-term use in chronic atrial fibrillation, to reduce the likelihood of systemic embolization. This particularly applies to patients with rheumatic heart disease and to prosthetic valve recipients. Those patients with a previous history of thrombo-embolism (stroke or TIA) and those who have a documented atrial thrombus, are also candidates for long-term anticoagulant therapy.

Table 44.3: Management of atrial fibrillation
• Heart-rate control
• Anticoagulation
• Electrical cardioversion
• Radiofrequency ablation

If the patient's clinical status is poor and hemodynamics are unstable, electrical cardioversion with 100 to 200 Joules of energy is the treatment of choice, in an attempt to restore sinus rhythm. There are two requisites before cardioversion is attempted. Firstly, the patient should not have received digitalis in the previous 48 hours. Digitalis not only decreases the threshold for defibrillation, but also predisposes to the risk of life-threatening arrhythmias. Secondly, an oral anti-coagulant should be initiated before cardioversion and continued for atleast four weeks. This is because atrial thrombi are more likely to dislodge as emboli, once sinus rhythm is restored. Cardioversion should not be attempted if there is a documented left atrial clot.

In patients who are symptomatic but either refractory or intolerant to several antiarrhythmic agents, the final option is of radiofrequency ablation (RFA). Advantages of RFA are not only freedom from symptoms but also avoidance of the toxic effects of antiarrhythmic drugs and the need to monitor anticoagulant therapy.

CASE
45

Ventricular Premature Beats

CASE PRESENTATION

A 72-year old man arrived at the emergency room with shortness of breath, palpitation, anorexia and vomiting. He had been repeatedly hospitalized over the past 6 months, because of congestive heart failure due to ischemic cardiomyopathy. The patient had sustained myocardial infarction twice and his left ventricular ejection fraction was 25%. During his previous admission a month back, frequent multifocal ventricular premature complexes (VPCs) were detected, for which amiodarone 200 mg daily was added to his ongoing therapy. His dose of frusemide was escalated from 40 mg to 60 mg per day because of worsening heart failure. He was also receiving digoxin 0.25 mg once a day, 6 days in a week.

On examination, the patient was restless, orthopneic and in respiratory distress. There was mild pallor and the extremities were cold and clammy. The pulse was rapid, irregular and low in volume, with a BP of 104/66 mm Hg. The JVP was raised 5 cm above the angle of Louis and there was edema over the ankles and lower legs. The lower border of the liver was felt 4 cm below the costal margin and ascites was present. Fine inspiratory crackles were heard over the bases of lung fields bilaterally. The cardiac apical impulse was diffuse and displaced towards the axilla. On auscultation, both S_3 and S_4 were audible, producing a summation gallop rhythm. A soft pansystolic murmur was also heard at the cardiac apex, that radiated towards the left axilla and scapula. A 12-lead ECG was obtained, with a long-strip recording of lead L_{II} (Fig. 45.1)

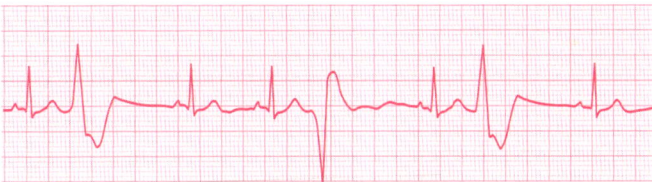

Figure 45.1: ECG showing multifocal ventricular premature beats

ECG INTERPRETATION

The ECG showed a fast irregular rhythm with frequent premature beats. The premature beats had a wide and bizarre QRS morphology, were not preceded by P waves, but were followed by a compensatory pause. The morphology of the premature beats, as well as the interval between the premature beat and the preceding sinus beat (coupling interval), were variable. At times, a very premature beat was superimposed upon the T wave of the preceding sinus beat. These findings are consistent with the diagnosis of multifocal ventricular premature complexes (VPCs) exhibiting the R-on-T phenomenon.

VPCs can be qualified on the basis of their pattern of occurrence and their location in the cardiac cycle. VPCs with an identical morphology and constant coupling interval are called unifocal VPCs. Those VPCs that have a variable morphology and changing coupling interval are called multifocal VPCs. That VPC which occurs late in the diastolic period of the preceding sinus beat (long coupling interval), just about when the next sinus beat is expected, is called an end-diastolic VPC. A VPC that is so premature (very short coupling interval) that it is superimposed upon the T wave of the preceding sinus impulse, is said to exhibit the R-on-T phenomenon. A VPC during a slow rhythm, that does not allow any sinus beat to be missed and is not followed by a compensatory pause, is called an interpolated VPC. VPCs alternating with sinus beats constitute a bigeminal rhythm (extrasystolic ventricular bigeminy). VPC after every two sinus beats represents trigeminy and a VPC after every third sinus beat constitutes a quadrigeminy. The degree of ventricular ectopy has been categorized as per the Lown's classification given in Table 45.1.

Table 45.1: Lown's classification of ventricular ectopy	
Category	**Degree of ectopy**
Class 0	No ectopy
Class 1	Less than 30/hour
Class 2	More than 30/hour
Class 3	Multiform VPCs
Class 4A	Couplets
Class 4B	Runs of 3 or more
Class 5	R-on-T phenomenon

CLINICAL DISCUSSION

Ventricular premature complexes (VPCs) can occur even in normal individuals, although they are more often due to organic heart disease. Causes of VPCs in normal persons are:
- Drugs e.g. beta-agonists, theophylline
- Emotional stress and physical exercise
- Smoking and high intake of tea/coffee
- Anxiety neurosis and thyrotoxicosis.

Cardiac conditions in which VPCs are observed are:

- Coronary Artery Disease
  Ischemia
  Infarction
  Reperfusion
- Congestive heart failure
  Hypertension
  Cardiomyopathy
  Ventricular aneurysm
- Mitral Valve Prolapse Syndrome
- Digitalis Treatment and Intoxication
- Cardiac Surgery and Catheterization.

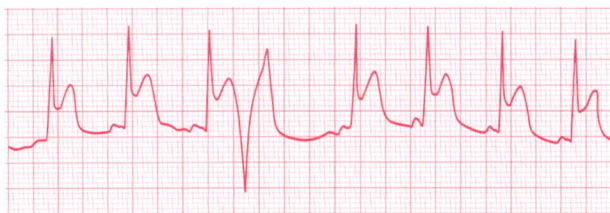

Figure 45.2: ECG showing a premature beat that exhibits the R-on-T phenomenon

A VPC that occurs very prematurely (very short coupling interval) super-imposes on the T wave of the preceding sinus beat and is said to exhibit the 'R-on-T' phenomenon (Fig. 45.2). This represents the occurrence of ventricular stimulation, during the vulnerable phase or the period of supernormal excitability and is likely to precipitate ventricular fibrillation. The 'R-on-T' phenomenon is observed in these situations:

- VPCs after acute myocardial infarction
- Very premature stimuli during external pacing
- Electrical cardioversion during digitalis therapy
- VPCs with underlying Q-T interval prolongation.

VPCs may be asymptomatic or associated with palpitation and a sensation of "missed beats". Awareness of VPCs is due to the post-VPC compensatory pause and increased force of contraction of the beat following the VPC. Neck pulsations may be felt due to atrial systole occurring with a closed tricuspid valve, since the atria and ventricles are activated almost synchronously.

MANAGEMENT ISSUES

The management of ventricular premature beats is governed by the severity of ectopy, symptoms of the patient and the presence of structural heart disease. Few isolated beats without symptoms and in the absence of heart disease are mostly left alone. If symptoms are present, causative factors need to be corrected. This includes alleviating anxiety, withdrawal of adrenergic drugs and reduction of smoking and beverage intake. If these measures do not suffice, beta-blockers are the drugs of choice to treat VPCs associated with anxiety, mitral valve prolapse and thyrotoxicosis.

VPCs occurring within 24 hours of myocardial infarction indicate reperfusion and carry a better prognosis than those that appear after 24 hours. Lidocaine and amiodarone are the drugs of choice to treat VPCs after myocardial infarction, heart surgery or after cardiac catheterization. Patients who have structural heart disease in the form of left ventricular hypertrophy (LVH), dilated cardiomyopathy (DCMP) or arrhythmogenic right ventricular dysplasia (ARVD), almost always deserve an antiarrhythmic drug such as amiodarone. When a patient of congestive heart failure on digitalis develops significant VPCs, it has to be decided on clinical grounds whether digitalis should be continued to manage the heart failure or withdrawn in view of drug intoxication. If digitalis is to be withdrawn, the antiarrhythmic drug of choice for digitalis induced VPCs is phenytoin sodium which should be used in conjunction with standard therapy of digitalis intoxication.

Antiarrhythmic drugs may be prescribed to control VPCs but before initiating treatment, the following issues need to be addressed:
- Aggravation of bradycardia and left ventricular dysfunction
- Proarrhythmic effects and likelihood of other tachyarrhythmias
- Potential systemic side-effects of long-term antiarrhythmic therapy
- Inappropriate drug usage, since the cause-and-effect relationship between VPCs and fatal arrhythmias has not been established.

Ventricular Tachycardia

CASE PRESENTATION

A 66-year old woman was brought to the emergency department with history of recurrent syncope preceded by palpitation and dizziness. She had sustained an anterior wall myocardial infarction 8 months back and also complained of exertional breathlessness with paroxysms of nocturnal dyspnea. She did not receive thrombolytic therapy and had not undergone primary angioplasty because she presented to the hospital, over 24 hours after the onset of chest pain. The patient was practically home-bound with limited physical activity and did not complain of exertional angina. An echocardiogram was performed a month after her myocardial infarction, which revealed a large wall motion abnormality involving the mid and distal septum, ventricular apex and the distal lateral wall. The left ventricular ejection fraction was 25%.

On examination, the patient was fully conscious and cooperative but tachypneic. The pulse was fast and irregular, low in volume, at a rate of 96 beats/min. with "missed beats". The BP was 110/66 mm Hg with a respiratory rate of 28/min. The JVP was not raised and there was no pitting edema over the ankles. The cardiac apical impulse was diffuse and displaced towards the axilla. Besides S_1 and S_2, an S_3 gallop sound was audible in early diastole. A soft holosystolic murmur was also heard at the cardiac apex. Bilateral basilar rales were audible over the lung fields. Along with a 12-lead ECG, a rhythm strip of lead L_{II} was obtained, which showed an alarming but transient abnormality (Fig. 46.1).

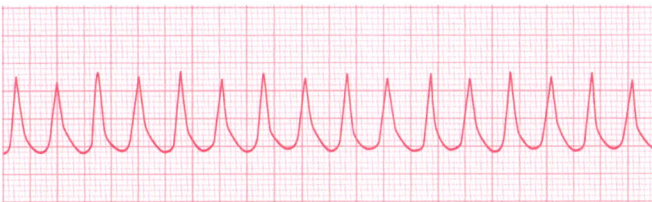

Figure 46.1: ECG strip showing monomorphic ventricular tachycardia

ECG INTERPRETATION

The ECG rhythm strip showed an abrupt onset of irregular tachycardia, at a rate of about 200 beats/min., with R-R interval of 7 to 8 mm. The QRS complexes were bizarre and wide, exceeding 0.14 sec in width, but did not conform to a bundle branch block pattern. The P and T waves were not discernable. These findings are consistent with the diagnosis of ventricular tachycardia. Ventricular tachycardia is due to enhanced automaticity of a latent ventricular pacemaker, that fires impulses rapidly. Alternatively, it is based on a closed re-entrant circuit around a fixed anatomical substrate in the ventricular myocardium (Fig. 46.2). Ventricular tachycardia may be sustained (lasting >30 sec) or non-sustained (lasting <30 sec). It is classified as monomorphic (similar QRS complexes) or polymorphic (variable QRS complexes) in nature.

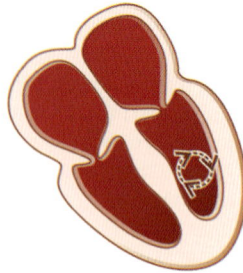

Figure 46.2: Diagram to illustrate ventricular re-entrant circuit

Polymorphic ventricular tachycardia is characterized by phasic variation of the QRS direction. A series of ventricular complexes are first up-pointing then down-pointing and this phenomenon occurs in a repetitive continuum (Fig. 46.3). Since this gives the appearance of rotation around the isoelectric line, it is called "Torsades de pointes", a ballet term which literally means "twisting around a point". Torsades de pointes is generally, associated with prolongation of the Q-T interval. The prolonged Q-T interval favours the occurrence of a ventricular premature beat that coincides with the T-wave of the preceding beat (R-on-T phenomenon) and initiates the ventricular tachycardia.

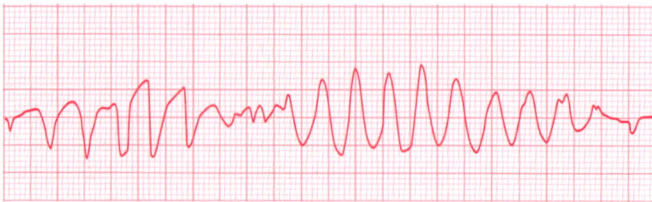

Figure 46.3: ECG showing polymorphic ventricular tachycardia

Ventricular tachycardia superficially resembles a supraventricular tachycardia conducted aberrantly to the ventricles. Features in favour of a supraventricular tachycardia are clock-like regularity, triphasic QRS morphology, normal QRS axis, stable hemodynamic parameters and response to carotid sinus massage.

CLINICAL DISCUSSION

A series of three or more successive ventricular ectopic beats constitutes a ventricular tachycardia. A ventricular tachycardia that lasts for more than 30 seconds and requires cardioversion for termination is called sustained ventricular tachycardia. A non-sustained ventricular tachycardia lasts for less than 30 seconds and ends spontaneously. Ventricular tachycardia is considered repetitive or recurrent if three or more discrete episodes are documented, while chronic ventricular tachycardia is that in which recurrent episodes occur for over a month. Sustained ventricular tachycardia (scar VT) is often based on structural heart disease wherein a fixed anatomical substrate facilitates a re-entrant mechanism. Causes of sustained ventricular tachycardia are:

- Myocardial scar
  Infarction
  Aneurysm
- Myocardial disease
  Myocarditis
  Cardiomyopathy
- Congestive failure
  Ischemic
  Hypertensive
- Valvular abnormality
  Mitral valve prolapse
  Rheumatic heart disease.

Symptoms due to ventricular tachycardia are palpitation because of fast heart rate and angina due to increased oxygen demand and shortened coronary filling time. Lack of atrio-ventricular synchrony can cause dyspnea (pulmonary edema) and syncope (low cardiac output). The hallmark of ventricular tachycardia is the dissociation between atrial systole and ventricular systole (A-V dissociation). On auscultation, the intensity of S_1 is variable because of changing diastolic filling period. Cannon *a* waves are observed in the neck veins due to atrial contraction against a closed tricuspid valve. An atrial impulse may occasionally find the ventricle receptive to depolarization and is able to "capture" the ventricle. A capture beat (complete capture) or a fusion beat (incomplete capture) is irrefutable evidence of A-V dissociation. Markers of electrical instability in survivors of acute myocardial infarction are:

- Documented ventricular arrhythmias on 24-hour Holter monitoring
- Reproducible tachycardia on programmed electrical stimulation (PES)
- Late depolarizations on signal averaged electrocardiogram (SAECG).

MANAGEMENT ISSUES

The management of ventricular tachycardia (VT) depends upon the etiology, the nature of heart disease and the hemodynamics of the patient. Ventricular tachycardia due to sympathetic stimulation (catecholaminergic VT), caused by stress, exercise or adrenergic drugs and in the absence of structural heart disease, responds well to beta-blockers. In the presence of heart disease and if hemodynamics are stable, chemical cardioversion with antiarrhythmic drugs is initiated. An intravenous bolus of lignocaine or amiodarone is followed by a maintenance infusion. Oral amiodarone is later continued indefinitely to prevent recurrence. Alternative agents are sotalol, propafenone, flecainide and ibutilide. If the hemodynamics are unstable due to hypotension, heart failure, or ongoing ischemia, electrical cardioversion with DC shock is the procedure of choice. An initial energy of 50 to 100 Joules is followed up with higher voltage, until sinus rhythm is restored. If there is circulatory shock to begin with, upto 360 Joules are used. Once sinus rhythm is restored, prophylactic pharmacological therapy is initiated and continued indefinitely.

The management of polymorphic ventricular tachycardia with Q-T prolongation is quite different. An infusion of magnesium sulphate or isoproterenol is used for chemical cardioversion. If the patient responds to beta-blockade, either long-term antiadrenergic therapy is initiated or cervical sympathetic ganglionectomy is offered. If the hemodynamics are unstable with hypotension or shock, electrical cardioversion is the procedure of choice, as per the protocol mentioned above. Alternatively, overdrive ventricular pacing is done, which is often successful. To patients with history of recurrent syncope or family history of sudden cardiac death (SCD) and to survivors of cardiac arrest, an implantable cardioverter defibrillator (ICD) device is offered.

Coronary Artery Disease

Chronic Stable Angina

CASE PRESENTATION

A 38-year old gentleman paid a visit to the cardiologist, with the complaint of retrosternal heaviness during brisk walking. The discomfort was described as a feeling of tightness in the chest and was associated with a sensation of suffocation and choking. The chest pain radiated towards the left shoulder, down the inner aspect of the left arm as well as to the neck and lower jaw. There was no history of dyspnea, palpitation, excessive sweating or syncope. The discomfort typically occurred when the patient undertook any form of physical activity, soon after a meal. He denied any chest pain at rest or during sleep. The frequency and severity of his episodic chest discomfort had not increased over the last three months. The patient was not taking any cardiovascular medication and had never undergone a blood glucose or lipid analysis. He smoked about 8 to 10 cigarettes a day for the last 20 years and took 5 to 6 alcoholic drinks over weekends. He did not follow any particular diet plan or exercise regime. His executive job entailed long hours of working and caused considerable mental stress. There was history of premature coronary artery disease as well as of diabetes mellitus, in several of his family members.

On examination, the patient was alert and in no distress. He was modestly overweight with a body mass index (BMI) of 27kg/m². The pulse rate was 84 beats/min. with a BP of 134/82 mm Hg and there were no signs of heart failure. Findings on general examination were xanthelasma on the upper eyelids, arcus senilis around the cornea and acanthosis nigricans over the nape of neck. The precordium was unremarkable with a normally located apex beat. There was no S_3 or S_4 gallop, murmur or friction rub upon auscultation. The lung fields were clear without any rhonchi or crepts. An ECG was obtained (Fig. 47.1).

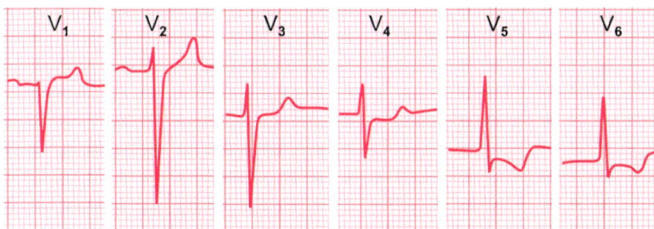

Figure 47.1: ECG showing S-T segment depression with T wave inversion in the lateral chest leads

ECG INTERPRETATION

The ECG showed normal sinus rhythm with normal P wave morphology and no prolongation of the P-R interval or Q-T interval. The QRS complexes were narrow, without significant Q waves or attenuation of the R wave height. A 2 mm horizontal depression of the S-T segment was observed in leads V_4, V_5 and V_6. The T wave was also inverted in leads V_5 and V_6. These findings are consistent with the diagnosis of lateral wall myocardial ischemia, a common feature in a patient who has angina pectoris.

Coronary artery disease is the most important cause of S-T segment depression. The degree of S-T segment depression (greater than 1 mm) correlates with the severity of coronary insufficiency. Besides being depressed, the morphology of the S-T segment, with increasing severity of myocardial ischemia, can be classified as shown in Figure 47.2.

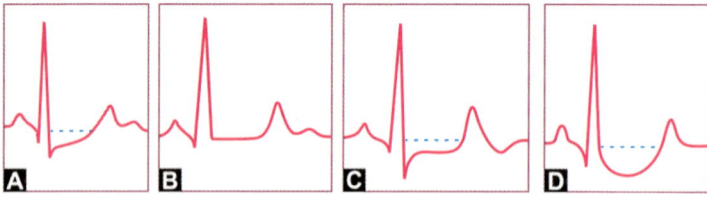

Figure 47.2: Nature of S-T segment depression with increasing severity of ischemia

A. Isolated J point depression (upsloping S-T segment)
B. Horizontality of S-T segment (sharp ST-T junction)
C. Plane S-T depression (horizontal S-T depression)
D. Sagging depression (hammock-like S-T segment).

Depression of the S-T segment constitutes the most useful criterion for the positivity of the stress ECG test, performed by exercising on a treadmill or bicycle ergometer. The degree of positivity of the stress test (mild, moderate or severe) can be gauged from several parameters of S-T segment depression. The magnitude of S-T segment depression and its shape are associated with the severity of coronary artery disease. Additionally, early appearance of S-T depression in the exercise period and longer persistence into the recovery period correlate with the positivity of the stress test.

Angina pectoris is described as a feeling of retrosternal heaviness or tightness, with a sensation of suffocation or choking. The pain is of a crushing or squeezing nature along with restlessness, sweating, palpitation, shortness of breath or extreme weakness. The pain may radiate to both shoulders and arms, down the inner aspect of left arm or to the neck and lower jaw. In contrast, the pain arising from the musculo-skeletal system of the chest is described as a dull ache or a sharp pricking sensation. The pain increases on deep inspiration, turning to one side, or on bending forwards. The pattern of radiation and accompaniments that characterize angina pectoris, are typically absent in muscular chest pain.

Stable angina is caused by an imbalance between the supply of and demand for oxygenated blood to the myocardium. The commonest cause is obstructive coronary artery disease due to atherosclerosis. Stable angina is due to coronary occlusion by one or more atherosclerotic plaques that have a small lipid core, a thick fibrous cap and are less prone to rupture. Conventional risk factors for coronary disease are advanced age, male sex, being overweight, tobacco abuse, diabetes mellitus, hypertension, hyperlipdemia, sedentary lifestyle, psychosocial stress and family history of coronary artery disease (Table 47.1).

Table 47.1: Conventional risk factors for coronary artery disease	
• Male Sex	• Hypertension
• Advanced age	• Hyperlipidemia
• Being overweight	• Diabetes mellitus
• Tobacco abuse	• Sedentary lifestyle
• Family history	• Psychosocial stress

Besides atherosclerotic coronary artery disease, there are some other atypical and uncommon causes of angina pectoris, which too cause an imbalance between myocardial oxygen supply and demand. These uncommon causes of angina are given in Table 47.2.

Table 47.2: Atypical causes of angina pectoris
Non-cardiac • Severe anemia • Thyrotoxicosis
Vascular • Coronary artery spasm • Microvascular disease
Cardiac • Aortic valve stenosis • Hypertensive heart disease • Hypertrophic cardiomyopathy

MANAGEMENT ISSUES

The first step in the management of stable angina pectoris is suitable life-style modification and control of cardiovascular risk factors. Patients should be advised to cut-down on calorie-dense foods, follow a regular exercise regimen, to quit smoking and manage psycho-social stress. Major risk factors such as hypertension, diabetes and hyperlipidemia should be treated with suitable drugs, in addition to correction of life-style.

Glyceryl trinitrate (GTN) is used sub-lingually for rapid relief from angina, while long-acting isosorbide mononitrate (ISMN) is given for long-term prophylaxis. Beta-blockers are the mainstay of therapy, as they reduce the rate and force of cardiac contraction and therefore the workload and oxygen demand.

In the scenario of beta-blocker contraindication or intolerance, a rate-limiting calcium antagonist like verapamil or diltiazem is used. Metabolic agents like nikorandil and trimetazidine are sometimes used. Low-dose aspirin prevents thrombotic events. If the patient is allergic or intolerant to aspirin, clopidogrel is employed. All patients should receive a statin, irrespective of their cholesterol level. Statins have amply proven their worth in preventing cardiovascular events. The ACE-inhibitor ramipril has also been shown to reduce CV events and all-cause mortality in patients with cardiovascular disease.

RECENT ADVANCES

Besides the conventional risk factors of coronary artery disease, certain new risk factors have been recently identified (Table 47.3). These include high levels of C-reactive protein (CRP), homocysteine (Hcy), lipoprotein (a) [Lp (a)], and fibrinogen (Fgn). However, the INTERHEART study clearly showed that majority of heart attacks across the globe can be conveniently explained on the basis of conventional risk factors. Modest intake of alcohol with high intake of fruits and vegetables were found to be important "anti-risk" factors.

Ranolazine is a new metabolically active agent used for the treatment of stable angina. Ivabradine is a recently introduced drug for heart-rate control, in patients who cannot tolerate uptitration of beta-blocker dose.

Table 47.3: Non-conventional risk factors for coronary artery disease
• C-reactive protein (CRP)
• Lipoprotein (a) [Lp(a)]
• Homocysteine (Hcy)
• Fibrinogen (Fgen)

CASE

48

Acute Coronary Syndrome

CASE PRESENTATION

A 56-year old gentleman was brought to the emergency department by his wife, in the wee hours of the morning. The man had complained of severe central chest pain with profuse sweating, during sexual intercourse. He was a known case of diabetes mellitus and hypertension. However, he was irregular with his medication and did not follow-up with his doctor periodically. The patient had not undergone a blood lipid analysis despite advice from his doctor and persistent request by his wife. He had a sedentary life-style and was on no particular dietary restrictions. He smoked 8 to 10 cigarettes everyday and took 3 to 4 pegs of whiskey, on most days of the week. A treadmill test performed one year earlier had been inconclusive, because the patient had failed to achieve the target heart rate. Recently, he had been complaining of frequent episodes to restlessness and belching, which he attributed to acidity and indigestion.

On examination, the patient was tachypneic and diaphoretic. He was markedly overweight with a body mass index (BMI) of about 32 kg/m^2. The pulse was irregular and low in volume with "skipped" beats. The extremities were cold and clammy. His heart rate was 104 beats/min. with a BP of 104/74 mm Hg. Skin tags and acanthosis nigricans were seen at the nape of the neck and xanthelasma were observed over the upper eyelids. The precordium and apex beat were unremarkable. The S$_1$ and S$_2$ were loud with a S$_3$ gallop; no murmur was audible. Few basilar rales were heard over the lung fields bilaterally. An ECG was obtained (Fig. 48.1).

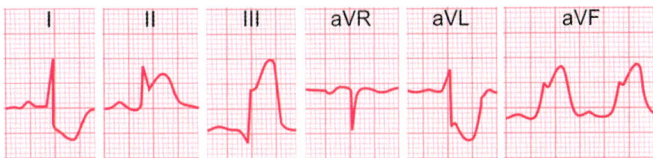

Figure 48.1: ECG showing S-T segment elevation in inferior leads with S-T segment depression in lateral leads

ECG INTERPRETATION

The ECG showed sinus rhythm with normal P waves and no prolongation of the Q-T interval. There was a 5 mm elevation of the S-T segment in leads L_{II}, L_{III} and avF. There was also S-T segment depression (reciprocal changes) in leads L_I and avL. There was no attenuation of the R wave or appearance of significant Q waves. These findings are consistent with the diagnosis of hyperacute phase of inferior wall myocardial infarction.

The phases of acute myocardial infarction are divided into hyperacute phase (0 hr to 6 hrs), recent phase (7 hrs to 7 days), evolved phase (8 days to 28 days) and stabilized phase (more than 29 days). In the hyperacute phase, the S-T segment is markedly elevated, which blends with the proximal limb of the tall T wave. In the evolved phase, the S-T segment elevation begins to settle down, T waves get inverted and Q waves appear. In the stabilized phase, there is normalization of the S-T segment and T waves but the Q waves persist (Fig. 48.2).

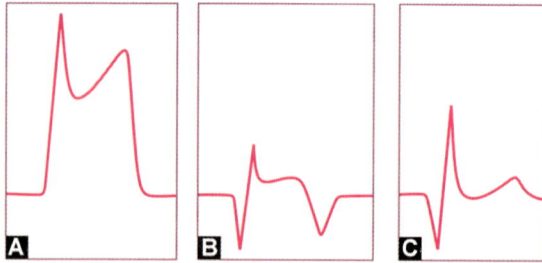

Figure 48.2: Diagram to illustrate the various phases of S-T elevation myocardial infarction

Myocardial infarction due to coronary occlusion, consists of a central necrotic core surrounded by a zone of injury and skirted by a water-shed area of ischemia. These areas form the pathological basis of the ECG changes observed in myocardial infarction. Q wave represents necrosis, S-T elevation is due to injury and T wave inversion is indicative of myocardial ischemia (Fig. 48.3).

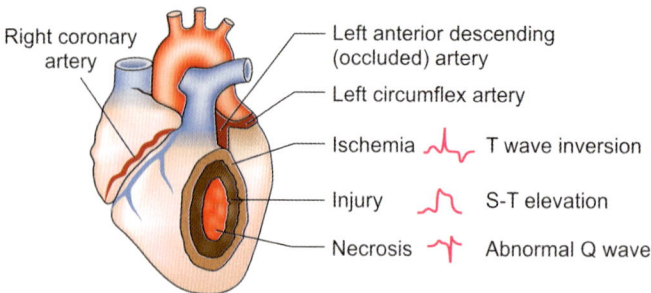

Figure 48.3: The pathological basis of ECG changes after acute myocardial infarction

The location of an infarct is identified from the particular ECG leads that show the classical findings of myocardial infarction (Table 48.1).

Table 48.1: Location of infarction from leads with Q waves	
Leads with Q waves	**Location of infarction**
V_1V_2	Septal
V_3V_4	Anterior
$V_5V_6L_1aVL$	Lateral
V_{1-4}	Anteroseptal
$V_{3-6}L_1aVL$	Anterolateral
$V_{1-6}L_1aVL$	Extensive anterior
L_1aVL	High lateral
$L_{II}L_{III}aVF$	Inferior

CLINICAL DISCUSSION

Acute coronary syndrome is classified into ST elevation myocardial infarction (STEMI), non-ST elevation myocardial infarction (NSTEMI) and unstable angina (UA). Since myocardial infarction (not angina) involves tissue necrosis, the levels of cardiac enzymes (creatine kinase and troponin), are elevated. The distinction between unstable angina and NSTEMI is therefore based on the cardiac enzyme levels. STEMI is also referred to as Q wave or transmural MI. NSTEMI is also designated as non-Q or subendocardial MI. This classification has therapeutic as well as prognostic implications. Acute coronary syndrome is due to coronary occlusion by an atherosclerotic plaque, which has a large lipid core, a thin fibrous cap and is more prone to rupture. A thrombus forms over the ruptured vulnerable plaque.

In variant angina, which is also known as Prinzmetal's angina, the basis of myocardial ischemia is not coronary thrombosis but arterial spasm. In an ischemic episode of vasospastic angina, the ECG changes are similar to those of hyperacute phase of infarction with S-T segment elevation and tall T waves. The difference is that the ECG changes do not evolve serially but settle down rapidly. Q wave never appear and levels of cardiac enzymes are not raised as there is no myocardial necrosis.

Myocardial infarction is classified on the basis of the age of infarct (recent or stabilized), site of infarct (anterior or inferior wall) and type of infarct (transmural or subendocardial). There may paucity of ECG findings if the infarction is small, atrial, posterior in location, or right ventricular MI. ECG findings of infarction are difficult to interpret in the presence of left bundle branch block, left ventricular hypertrophy, WPW syndrome and digoxin therapy. Reasons for a disparity between ECG changes and the clinical findings are left circumflex disease, hibernating myocardium, attenuation phenomenon or the presence of a mechanical complication.

Table 48.2: Types of regional wall motion

- Normal motion: full inward motion
- Hypokinesia:<50% inward motion
- Akinesia: no inward wall motion
- Dyskinesia: outward movement
- Aneurysmal: outpouching of wall.

On echocardiography, the systolic inward motion of the infarcted myocardial segment is reduced in extent, altogether absent or may even be paradoxically outward. The regional wall motion abnormality can be classified as given in Table 48.2. From the location of the regional wall motion abnormality (RWMA), it is possible to identify the coronary artery which is occluded (Fig. 48.4).

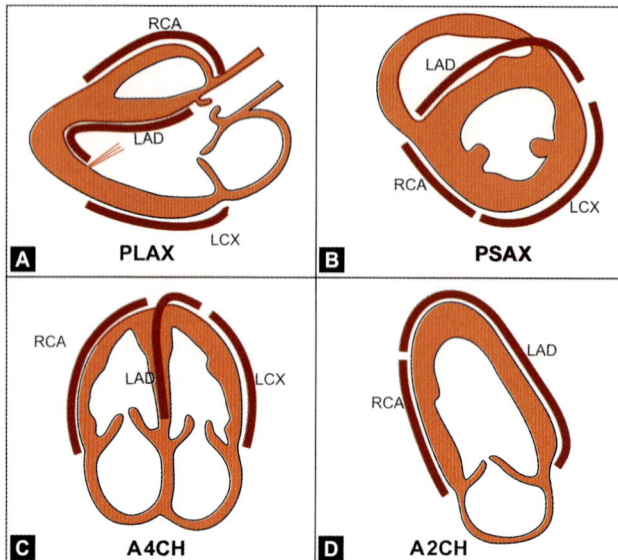

Figure 48.4: Identification of the occluded coronary artery from the location of wall motion abnormality
PLAX: Parasternal long axis; PSAX: Parasternal short axis; RCA: Right coronary artery; LAD: Left anterior descending artery; LCX: Left circumflex artery

MANAGEMENT ISSUES

All patients with an acute coronary syndrome (ACS), should ideally be managed in a coronary care unit (CCU), where the speed of instituting treatment improves myocardial salvage (time is muscle). The long-term survival after myocardial infarction heavily depends upon the extent of myocardial salvage (muscle is time). The essentials of treatment are bed-rest, oxygen, opiate analgesia, aspirin

162.5 mg stat and clopidogrel 300 mg stat. Patient of STEMI may be taken up for percutaneous coronary intervention (PCI), if there is rapid access to a Cath-Lab facility. If not, the patient should receive thrombolytic therapy, provided there are no contraindications.

Patient of NSTEMI should receive heparin, nitrate and a beta-blocker. High risk patients are taken up for coronary angiography with revascularization. Coronary artery revascularization is undertaken by percutaneous transluminal coronary angioplasty (PTCA) or by coronary artery bypass graft (CABG) surgery. PTCA is suitable for significant (>70% stenosis) single-vessel disease or 2-vessel disease. CABG is preferable for 3-vessel disease, 2-vessel disease including proximal LAD and left main-stem occlusion.

RECENT ADVANCES

A number of scoring systems have been developed, to risk-stratify patients presenting with an acute coronary syndrome. The most commonly used is the TIMI (Thrombolysis In Myocardial Infarction) Risk score, that was derived from trials of low molecular weight heparin. The TIMI system assigns a binary score (0 or 1) to seven independent risk factors, which have a similar predictive value. Higher the score, greater is the risk of death or recurrent ischemia at 14 days. The seven risk factors of the TIMI score, are given in Table 48.3.

Table 48.3: TIMI risk score after acute coronary syndrome
• Sixty-five years of age or older
• Three or more CV risk factors
• Significant coronary stenoses
• S-T segment deviation, > 2 mm
• Use of aspirin prior to admission
• Two or more anginal episodes within previous 24 hours
• Elevated cardiac enzyme levels (creatine kinase or troponin)

49

Papillary Muscle Rupture

CASE PRESENTATION

A 63-year old woman was wheeled into the emergency room, with the complaints of vague chest discomfort, profuse sweating and sinking sensation lasting about 5 hours. She also had retching and vomiting for which she took some antacid, thinking that it was "gas-trouble". When there was no relief, the patient's daughter deemed it necessary to get an ECG done. The ECG findings were alarming and therefore she was admitted to the coronary care unit (CCU). There she received thrombolytic therapy and remained stable for the next 3 days. On the 4th day of her admission, she felt breathless and was unable to lie flat in bed. There was no fresh chest pain and the cardiac monitor did not show any serious arrhythmia, except for an occasional ventricular premature complex.

On examination, the patient was tachypneic, diaphoretic and appeared to be in distress. She looked pale and her extremities were cold and clammy. The pulse was fast, irregular and of low volume, with a rate of 104 beats/min. Her BP was 106/74 mm Hg in the right arm and the respiratory rate was 28/min. The JVP was not raised and there was no edema over the ankles. The precordium was hyperkinetic and the cardiac apex beat was displaced towards the left axilla. The S_1 and S_2 were normal but an S_3 gallop sound was appreciated in diastole. A soft systolic murmur was audible over the cardiac apex. The murmur radiated towards the axilla and could be heard upto the left scapula. Bilateral coarse crackles were heard over the lung fields.

ECG showed sinus tachycardia with 5 mm elevation of the S-T segment in leads L_{II}, L_{III} and aVF. There was reciprocal S-T segment depression in leads L_I and aVL. These findings were consistent with the diagnosis of hyperacute inferior wall myocardial infarction (Fig. 49.1). Additionally, there was elevation of the S-T segment in the right-sided chest leads V_3R and V_4R. This was indicative of right ventricular infarction.

ECHO revealed a normal sized left ventricle with an ejection fraction of 45%. There was dilatation of the right ventricle and right atrium. The postero-basal segment of the left ventricle and free wall of the right ventricle were hypokinetic. There was no mass or thrombus in any chamber. The posterior leaflet of the mitral valve exhibited an exaggerated whip-like motion (Fig. 49.2). The tip moved past the mitral annular plane and deep into the left atrium. It failed to coapt with the anterior leaflet at the end of diastole. On colour flow mapping, an eccentric jet was seen in the left atrium, that was directed towards the posterior left atrial wall. These findings are consistent with the diagnosis of flail mitral leaflet due to papillary muscle rupture.

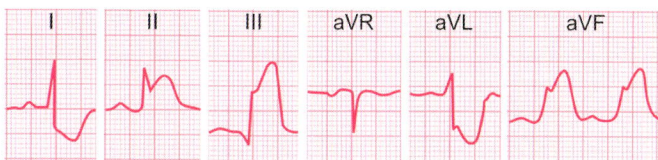

Figure 49.1: ECG showing the hyperacute phase of inferior wall myocardial infarction

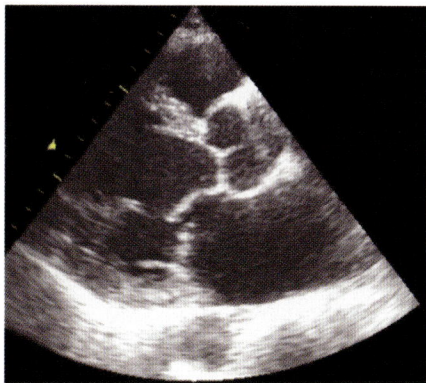

Figure 49.2: ECHO showing exaggerated motion of a flail posterior mitral leaflet

CLINICAL DISCUSSION

Acute mitral regurgitation (MR) in a setting of acute myocardial infarction, occurs either due to papillary muscle rupture or because of papillary muscle dysfunction. Rupture of a papillary muscle due to ischemic necrosis causes a flail mitral valve leaflet (Fig. 49.3). Since rupture of the postero-medial papillary muscle is more common than that of the antero-lateral muscle, often it is the posterior mitral leaflet (PML) that is flail. It generally follows inferior wall infarction due to occlusion of the posterior descending branch of the right coronary artery. Papillary muscle dysfunction is due to ischemic restriction of papillary function or akinesia of the infero-basal wall that does not adequately shorten in systole. As

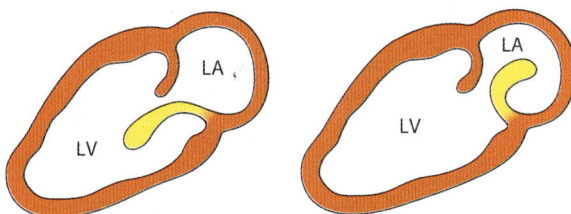

Figure 49.3: Diagram to illustrate whip-like motion of a flail posterior mitral leaflet
LV: Left ventricle; LA: Left atrium

a result, the posterior mitral leaflet fails to reach the plane of the valve annulus and the coaptation point of mitral leaflets is distally located into the left ventricle.

In acute MR due to myocardial infarction (MI), the left ventricular (LV) systolic function often remains unimpaired. In pump failure due to extensive MI, there is severe LV dysfunction. Although there is no time for left ventricular dilatation to develop, an acute rise in left ventricular end-diastolic pressure (LVEDP) rapidly produces frank pulmonary edema. The systolic murmur of acute MR is short and soft compared to the long and loud murmur of MR due to chronic valvular disease. This is because of two reasons. Firstly, the large mitral orifice created by acute MR, does not generate much turbulence across the valve. Secondly, the rapid rise in left atrial pressure and decline in pressure gradient impedes regurgitation, during the later half of systole. Besides papillary muscle rupture due to myocardial infarction, other causes of acute mitral regurgitation are blunt trauma to the chest wall and valve dehiscence in case of infective endocarditis (Table 49.1). Another cause of a systolic murmur after myocardial infarction is ventricular septal rupture.

Table 49.1: Causes of acute mitral regurgitation
• Myocardial infarction
• Infective endocarditis
• Chest wall trauma

On Doppler or on color flow mapping, the MR flow velocity or color jet is eccentric and directed towards the posterior left atrial wall (Fig. 49.4). The jet area may be much less than the actual amount of MR; hence there is a risk of underestimating the severity of acute MR. The flail leaflet of papillary muscle rupture resembles the floppy leaflet of mitral valve prolapse with subtle differences. The prolapsing leaflet just buckles but does not flap freely and it enters the left atrium only for a brief period (Table 49.2).

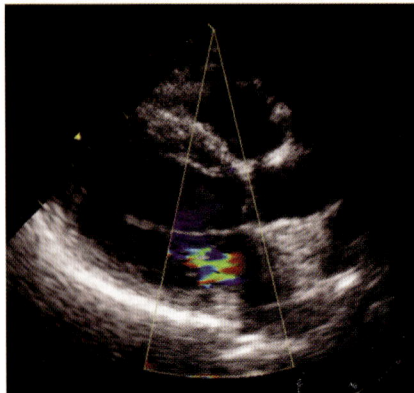

Figure 49.4: ECHO showing an eccentric jet of mitral regurgitation

Table 49.2: Differences between flail mitral leaflet and mitral valve prolapse		
	Flail leaflet	**Prolapsed leaflet**
Range of motion	flaps freely	just buckles
Entry into left atrium extent duration	 deep into for long time	 just enters for short time
Direction of tip	towards LA	towards LV

MANAGEMENT ISSUES

Mitral regurgitation due to coronary heart disease is multifactorial and papillary muscle dysfunction or rupture is one of the causes. Other reasons are dysfunctional ventricular remodelling with increased sphericity and mitral annular dilatation due to ventricular enlargement. Medical management includes vasodilators along with a diuretic, provided the blood pressure allows their use. In surgical treatment, since the valvular anatomy is generally not distorted, mitral valve replacement is not the answer. Instead restrictive annuloplasty, which involves insertion of an undersized ring to improve leaflet apposition, is preferable. Moreover, annuloplasty preserves left ventricular geometry and spares the patient from the problems of anticoagulation (thrombosis, bleeding and monitoring).

CASE
50

Left Ventricular Aneurysm

CASE PRESENTATION

A 68-year old man came with his son to his treating cardiologist, for a periodic heart check-up. Three months back, the patient has sustained an anterior wall myocardial infarction (MI), for which he was treated in this very hospital. At that time, he received oral aspirin, sub-cutaneous enoxaparin and an infusion of nitroglycerine. He was not given thrombolytic therapy because he presented over 24 hours after the onset of his chest pain and Q waves had already appeared on the ECG. The patient also declined coronary angiography, because he was not ready to undergo a revascularization procedure. Thereafter, he did not develop post-MI angina, but he did complain of some fatigue and exertional breathlessness.

On examination, the patient was tachypneic while lying on the couch in the doctor's chamber. The pulse rate was 96 beats/min. with a BP of 110/74 mm Hg over the right arm. The JVP was not raised and there was no edema over the ankles. The precordium was remarkable because of a prominent bulge and a double apical impulse. The apex beat was diffuse and sustained and extended medially and upwards, upto the 3rd intercostal space. On auscultation, the S_1 and S_2 were normal but a soft S_3 sound was audible in early diastole. No murmur or pericardial friction rub was appreciated. The breath sounds were vesicular with few crepitations audible over the lower lung fields.

ECG showed attenuation of R waves in the antero-septal precordial leads. There was coving and elevation of the S-T segment with inversion of the T waves (Fig. 50.1). The cardiac Troponin -T test was negative. X-ray chest findings were increased cardio-thoracic ratio with a large bulge on the left border of the heart. An arc-like hemispherical calcification was seen within the bulge (Fig. 50.2).

ECHO revealed a dilated left ventricle with an ejection fraction of 35%. There was a large dyskinetic area involving the mid and distal interventricular septum as well as the left ventricular apex. The dyskinetic area underwent outward systolic expansion with a persistent deformity during diastole. The wall of the dyskinetic area was more echogenic than the adjacent myocardium. A laminated mass was observed contiguous with the dyskinetic area, with which it moved synchronously (Fig. 50.3). These findings are consistent with the diagnosis of left ventricular aneurysm with mural thrombus.

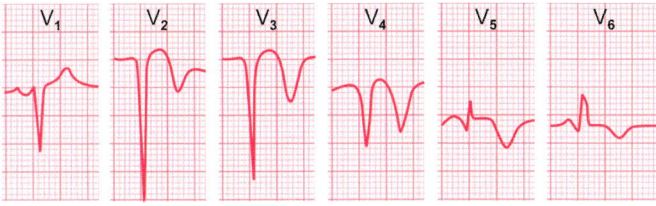

Figure 50.1: ECG showing R wave attenuation,
S-T coving and T wave inversion

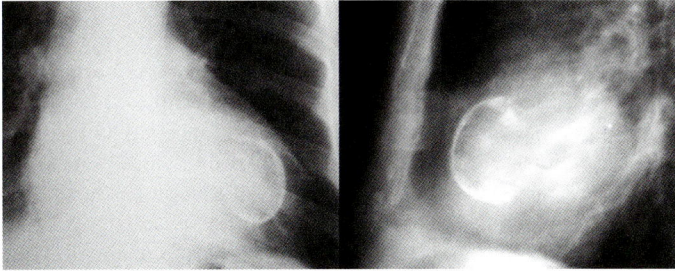

Figure 50.2: X-ray showing an arc-like calcification within a ventricular bulge

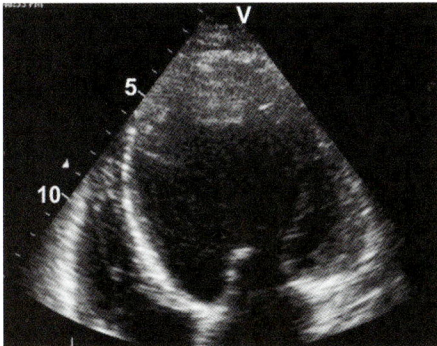

Figure 50.3: ECHO showing a mural thrombus
arising from the ventricular apex

CLINICAL DISCUSSION

A ventricular aneurysm usually develops after an anterior wall myocardial infarction, due to occlusion of the left anterior descending coronary artery. It rarely follows inferior wall infarction. On ECG, if the typical pattern of evolved myocardial infarction (MI) persists for three or more months after acute MI, ventricular aneurysm should be suspected. On precordial inspection, the ventricular aneurysm produces a double left ventricular apical impulse. If the aneurysm is particularly large, it causes a sustained and diffuse apical impulse that extends medially and upwards, by two or more intercostal spaces.

Table 50.1: Differences between true LV aneurysm and Pseudo-aneurysm		
	LV aneurysm	**Pseudo-aneurysm**
Shape	Wide neck	Narrow neck
Location	Apex of LV	Posterior wall
Motion	Dyskinetic	Expansile
Wall	Myocardium	Pericardium
Rupture	Unlikely	Liable
Thrombus	Laminar	Fills cavity

A ventricular aneurysm is a large bulge-like deformity with a wide neck, located at or near the apex of the left ventricle. It is more common after damage to the anterior wall than after inferior wall infarction. The aneurysm exhibits dyskinesia or outward systolic expansion and a persistent deformity during diastole. The wall of the aneurysm is made of myocardium and is more echogenic than adjacent areas because it is made of fibrous scar tissue. It does not rupture but is often associated with a pedunculated or laminated ventricular thrombus.

A false aneurysm (pseudo-aneurysm) follows rupture of the left ventricular free wall, where the resultant hemopericardium clots and seals the breach by pericardial adhesions. The neck of the pseudo-aneurysm that communicates with the left ventricle is narrower than the aneurysm itself. The pseudo-aneurysm appears as a globular extracardiac pouch. A false aneurysm is located on the posterolateral LV wall and is more common after inferior wall than after anterior wall infarction. It is not expansile and remains constant in size. The wall of the aneurysm is made of pericardium and it is less echogenic than adjacent areas. It is friable, more liable to rupture and it is often filled with a thrombus caused by hemopericardium. The differences between a true aneurysm and a pseudo-aneurysm are given in Table 50.1.

The development of a left ventricular aneurysm after acute myocardial infarction is a serious complication. Most patients go on to develop intractable congestive heart failure requiring aggressive decongestive therapy. There is a higher likelihood of ventricular tachycardia originating from the myocardial scar. The incidence of post-infarction unstable angina is also increased. Moreover, fragments of the mural thrombus in the aneurysmal pouch may dislodge to produce distal embolism (Table 50.2).

Table 50.2: Complications of ventricular aneurysm
• Recurrent ventricular tachycardia
• Post-MI unstable angina pectoris
• Intractable congestive heart failure
• Mural thrombus with distal embolism

MANAGEMENT ISSUES

Presence of a thrombus within a ventricular aneurysm is an established indication for oral anticoagulant therapy. Other definite indications for anticoagulation are mechanical prosthetic valve and left atrial thrombus with mitral stenosis. While it takes 3 to 5 days for the therapeutic effect of an oral anticoagulant like warfarin to take over, heparin is given in this interim period. Unfractionated heparin requires monitoring of prothrombin time (PT) and aPTT, but it is cost-effective. Low molecular weight heparin (LMWH) like enoxaparin is more expensive but does not require monitoring.

It is established practice to prescribe aspirin, a statin, an ACE-inhibitor and a beta-blocker to every survivor of myocardial infarction, unless there is a specific contraindication. A diuretic is added to reduce cardiac workload, if there are symptoms of pulmonary congestion. An aldosterone antagonist like spironolactone or eplerenone can reduce cardiac workload and improve ventricular remodelling. A nitrate is prescribed for post-infarction angina while amiodarone is used if serious ventricular arrhythmias are documented.

It is not uncommon for patients who develop a ventricular aneurysm, to have left main or triple-vessel coronary artery disease (TVD). Resection of the aneurysm can be contemplated at the time of coronary artery bypass grafting (CABG) surgery which is performed for either unstable angina or for refractory heart failure.

Index

Page numbers followed by *f* refer to figure and *t* refer to table, respectively.